MW01092596

Drug Metabolism in Psychiatry

A Clinical Guide

Daniel J. Carlat, MD
Publisher and Editor-in-Chief
The Carlat Psychiatry Report

Third Edition

Drug Metabolism in Psychiatry:
A Clinical Guide

Copyright © 2015 by Daniel J. Carlat, MD. All rights reserved.

ISBN # 978-0-692-35788-0

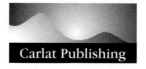

Carlat Publishing

Published by *Carlat Publishing, LLC*

P.O. Box 626, Newburyport, MA 01950

Ordering Information:

Online at www.TheCarlatReport.com
Call 866-348-9279
Write *The Carlat Psychiatry Report*, P.O. Box 626, Newburyport, MA 01950

Acknowledgements

This book is dedicated to my children, Ari and Sophia, and to my wife, Tammy.

For invaluable assistance, I also want to acknowledge:

- Paul Carlat, MD, a wonderful father and psychiatrist, who test-drove the book in his own practice, and let me know when something just didn't make sense.

- Marcia Zuckerman, MD, an editorial board member of *The Carlat Psychiatry Report* and quite possibly the most talented person on earth at making medical prose both relevant and comprehensible.

Table of Contents

Appendix

Tables and Charts

Preface

Really understanding the complex world of drug metabolism can be enormously tedious, and is something that few of us want to spend much time doing. Making the task even more difficult, many of us are skeptical that knowing all this stuff will really make much of a difference in our clinical practice.

I used to be a skeptic. I thought most of the ink spent on drug interactions was motivated by drug companies looking to find a niche for their drugs in a competitive market. But over time, I have become a convert to the value of really understanding basic drug metabolism concepts.

Here are some examples from my own clinical practice:

- A patient has panic attacks and needs relief more quickly than is provided by swallowing an Ativan (lorazepam) tablet. Knowing that sublingual absorption bypasses the liver and goes directly to the heart, I recommend she put the Ativan under her tongue, which provides her relief within 10 minutes.

- A patient on lithium is diagnosed with chronic hepatitis. He wonders if his lithium dose has to be adjusted. Knowing that lithium is not metabolized by the liver but is excreted unchanged by the kidneys, I assure him that the dose can remain the same, as long as his kidneys are healthy.

- A patient on Klonopin (clonazepam) has developed migraine headaches and tells me that her neurologist just started Tegretol (carbamazepine), and she has suffered more anxiety since then. She wonders if Tegretol might be causing her anxiety. Knowing that Tegretol is a strong inducer of various metabolic enzymes, I check my handy drug interactions chart and notice that it can decrease levels of Klonopin. I tell her this, and suggest she increase her Klonopin dose.

Basically, the more you know about the intricacies of drug metabolism, the more you will be in control of drug effects on your patients.

Here are eight specific ways that I hope you will be able to apply what you learn from this book to your clinical practice:

1. Knowledgeably discuss with your patients when they should take a specific drug on a full or an empty stomach.

2. Be able to confidently decide when it makes sense to prescribe an extended-release or transdermal version of a psychiatric drug, and when it's simply not worth the extra cost.

3. Understand the relationship between half-life and steady state, allowing you to roughly predict how much of a given drug is in your patient's bloodstream at any time—useful for knowing when to order levels and for determining dosing intervals.

4. Memorize the relatively few common and clinically relevant drug-drug interactions in psychiatry, and learn what to do with that information.

5. Understand the science of pharmacogenomics, and become an intelligent and skeptical consumer of genetic testing— most of which is not yet ready for prime time.

6. Understand how the kidney excretes drugs, thereby becoming a master prescriber of lithium.

7. Understand how monoamine oxidase inhibitors (MAOIs) may interact with foods and other medications.

8. Understand how generic medications may differ from their branded counterparts.

So, thank you very much for deciding to read what I have to say. If you see anything you particularly like or dislike in the following pages, please let me know by email (daniel.carlat@thecarlat report.com) or by phone at 866-348-9279. Your comments and criticisms will help me with future editions, and glowing words of praise will act as an effective mood enhancer, with a half-life of several hours at the least!

Preface to Third Edition

The first edition of this book was published in 2005, under the title "When Molecules Collide." We quickly ran out of copies, and in 2006 I added several chapters, and changed the name to "Drug Metabolism in Psychiatry"—not because that's catchy, but because some people thought the original title referred to a science fiction novel instead of a psychiatry textbook. We ran out of the 2006 edition long ago, but I delayed writing a new revision because I didn't think much had changed in the world of drug metabolism.

But by now, it's time for an update. In this edition I have added information about the newer antipsychotics and antidepressants, and I have downgraded my earlier optimism regarding the clinical utility of pharmacogenetic testing—10 years later, we are still waiting for a robust study proving that the testing actually improves our prescribing.

As with all of our Carlat Publishing products, my goal in making these revisions was to come closer to my ideal: a book that quickly answers practical clinical questions. I'll be curious to see what you think.

Sincerely,
Daniel J. Carlat, MD
Newburyport, Massachusetts
January 10, 2015

Section I

The Basics

Chapter 1

Introduction:
An Overview of Drug Metabolism

There are three phases of drug metabolism that you should learn about in order to enhance your skills as a psychopharmacologist.

1. **Absorption**, which refers to everything between your patient popping the pill in the mouth and the drug getting into the bloodstream.

2. **Distribution**, meaning getting the drug from the bloodstream to the tissue where it exerts its therapeutic effect, which, in the case of most psychiatric drugs, is the brain.

3. **Excretion**, meaning getting rid of the drug. This is the most important topic for us, and encompasses enzymatic breakdown, drug-drug interactions, half-lives, and the like.

Let's begin this journey with a very basic question: Why do we need drug metabolism at all?

The best thinking among pharmacologists is that metabolism started when early organisms realized that they could improve their chances of survival by producing toxins and delivering them to potential predators. While poisoning enemies was good fun, a problem arose: how to avoid poisoning yourself. Metabolic enzyme systems therefore initially evolved in order to get rid of these endogenous toxins. But they turned out to be quite good at neutralizing exogenous toxins, such as food by-products and (fast-forward a billion years) modern pharmaceuticals.

Drugs that enter our systems need to get into cells to work, and the very first thing that needs to happen to accomplish this is absorption (see **Chapter 2**). For absorption to happen, the stomach must grind down pills and capsules so that the molecules can come into contact with intestinal villi, where most of the actual absorption into the bloodstream takes place. To be absorbed, drugs have to cross fatty cell membranes, and they are fat-soluble in order to accomplish this task.

To effectively prescribe drugs, you should know a bit about *pharmacokinetics,* which is the study of how long drugs stick around inside the body, and what concentrations they typically achieve. The most clinically relevant parameters are *half-life* and *AUC* (area under the curve). The half-life is a measure of how rapidly half the amount of a drug is excreted, and the AUC represents the entire amount of drug that is present in the blood over a given period of time. **Chapter 3** focuses on half-life, steady state, and the whole field of pharmacokinetics.

The last few years have witnessed a great many "extended-release" (ER) formulations of old drugs. Obviously, a lot of this is marketing, since these new formulations tend to appear just as the "immediate-release" (IR) versions of the drugs are about to go off patent. But ER forms have their advantages at times. They typically allow once daily dosing and they usually cause fewer side effects, since the drugs don't get dumped into the system all at once. In **Chapter 4** we look specifically at how different ER drugs are packaged, and we look skeptically at whether they are really worth their high cost.

After drugs have worked their magic, we have to get rid of them. How do we accomplish this? The answer, which we discuss in **Chapter 5,** is that we transform them into water-soluble versions of themselves, so that they can be swept away in (watery) urine or stool. The main way we do this is via Cytochrome P450 enzymes and glucuronidation, which you'll learn about in the Chapter 5 as well.

In **Chapter 6** we go over some basic pharmacology and describe all the drug-drug interactions that psychiatrists should actually be concerned about.

In **Chapter 7** we review the ways in which aging changes drug metabolism, with an emphasis on prescribing for the elderly.

Chapter 8 tackles the often confusing topic of MAOI interactions, including a brief review of the selegiline patch (EMSAM).

In **Chapter 9** we provide a primer on generic drugs, and evaluate whether there are meaningful differences in bioavailability between generics and their brand name counterparts.

Chapter 10 is all about the kidney, that intimidating organ that we all know we should know more about but have been studiously avoiding, because it seems like such a momentous task. We show you that the kidney is made up of nephrons that do the work of drug excretion, and how understanding the dynamics of tubule absorption will help you feel very comfortable prescribing lithium and knowing when you need to order lithium levels.

We devote **Chapter 11** to the field of pharmacogenomics. We discuss the differences in how people metabolize certain drugs, we explain P450 genotyping, and we discuss whether there are patients in whom you should order such testing.

Finally, the **Appendix** brings the most useful charts and tables together for easy reference.

By the way, I didn't make all this stuff up. I've relied on several great books on pharmacology, which are listed and reviewed in my **Annotated (and Opinionated) Bibliography** at the end. In addition, I've scattered various relevant journal and website references throughout the text.

A Glossary of Drug Metabolism Terms

Here is a brief glossary of some of the more important terms used in this book for your referencing pleasure:

Absorption: Getting the drug from the mouth to the bloodstream

Distribution: Getting the drug from the bloodstream to the site of action

Excretion: Getting rid of the drug

Biotransformation: Chemically changing a drug so that it can be excreted

Cytochrome P450: A family of enzymes responsible for Phase I biotransformation

Glucuronidation: The addition of glucuronic acid to a drug, and the most common type of Phase II biotransformation

Substrate: The drug that is acted upon by metabolic enzymes

Inhibitor: A drug that interferes with an enzyme's ability to metabolize another drug

Inducer: A drug that stimulates the production of more metabolic enzymes

Slow metabolizer: A person who metabolizes drugs unusually slowly

Ultra-rapid metabolizer: A person who metabolizes drugs unusually quickly

Pharmacokinetics: What the body does to the drug

Pharmacodynamics: What the drug does to the body

Chapter 2

What Happens After You Swallow a Pill: Absorption

When a patient swallows a drug, it gets absorbed because the molecules are small enough to pass through cell membranes in the gut, and then into capillaries, which whisk them off to do their pharmacodynamic duties. Most drugs that we use are *lipophilic,* meaning that they have no ionic charge. Only lipophilic drugs diffuse easily through cell membranes in the gut and in the capillaries.

Oral drugs start out in our patients' mouths, but usually they spend so little time there before being swallowed that no absorption occurs. The main exception to this rule in psychiatry is sublingual administration of benzodiazepines, which we prescribe when we want to do something about a panic attack right away. Sublingual administration of Ativan (lorazepam) works somewhat faster than regular oral intake.

Why Do Sublingual Benzos Work Faster?

While the speed at which sublingual benzos are absorbed is not entirely clear, and has probably been exaggerated for marketing purposes, there are theoretically two reasons for a faster onset of action. First, and most obviously, the drug starts getting absorbed the second it is placed under the tongue, knocking off the several minutes required for it to move down the esophagus and into the stomach and small intestine. Second, drugs absorbed in most of the GI tract have to go into the "portal circulation." Blood vessels draining from the small intestine head directly into the liver, which begins the process of drug biotransformation even before the drug reaches the heart, and from there, the brain. This is famously known as the "first pass" effect, because drugs pass first through the liver *en route* to the heart. Depending on the drug, the liver may munch up well over 50% of the active ingredient before it has a chance to work anywhere in the body.

The two regions of the GI tract that bypass the greedy liver are the sublingual area and the rectal area. Thus, a benzodiazepine dissolving under the tongue takes the express train to the heart, and then to the brain, where it can work quickly — how quickly depends on the drug and other factors, such as how long your patient can refrain from swallowing the pill as it dissolves. Eventually, of course, the circulatory system will present it to the liver for its Shiatsu massage and degradation.

Where Does Most Absorption Actually Occur?

Assuming that the pill is swallowed, it then moves down the esophagus and into the stomach. For most of the drugs we prescribe, the stomach does very little absorption, and instead grinds and shoots acid at the tablet, helping it to disintegrate, so that the drug molecules can expose themselves to the gut wall and get absorbed. Most actual absorption doesn't occur until drugs reach the small intestine, an organ that is specialized for this task by folding itself into millions of villi and microvilli. My favorite small intestine factoid is that it would cover six football fields if completely flattened out. Now that's a lot of absorption.

Medications and the Annoying Stomach

Patients often want to know whether to take medications with meals or not. There are two parts to the answer: the first relates to comfort, the second to rate of absorption.

In terms of comfort, many patients experience nausea when they take psychiatric medications. For selective serotonin reuptake inhibitors (SSRIs), some of this comes from stimulation of serotonin receptors in the gut wall, a problem that won't go away by eating a snack with your Prozac. But there is also some local irritation, both with SSRIs and with other drugs, and taking medications with a meal often helps. I tell my patients with nausea from any drug to try taking their medication with food.

Of course, food does slow the rate of gastric emptying, and some drugs are absorbed marginally faster on an empty stomach. If nausea is not a problem, I tell patients to take those drugs with plenty of water (to speed transit) and without food.

Interestingly, though, some drugs are absorbed more effectively *with* food, for reasons that are not entirely clear. Zoloft (sertraline), for example, is absorbed *faster* after a meal, and the maximum concentration is actually *increased* by 25% when taken with food. By contrast, while Geodon (ziprasidone) and Latuda (lurasidone) are not absorbed faster with food, they are more fully absorbed, so that their blood levels are two to three times higher when taken with a meal. One theory proposed to explain this is that Geodon capsules require extra acid to dissolve into absorbable form, and what better way to provide that acid than to stimulate its production with food?

Food and the Erectile Dysfunction Drugs

The effect of meals on absorption is most famous in the case of the phosphodiesterase (PDE5) inhibitors Viagra (sildenafil) and Levitra (vardenafil). We have the most complete data for Viagra, whose absorption is delayed by an hour if taken with a "high fat" meal. Any meal will delay its absorption to some extent, but your pizza-type meals will delay gastric emptying profoundly while the stomach is savoring those five different types of cheeses. Absorption is not only delayed, but is actually reduced by food, with maximum plasma concentration being decreased by about 30%. That's certainly enough to put a dent in its efficacy.

Practical advice for patients? Waiting a good hour or two after meals is the best strategy, but if they *must* eat right away, having them take a *higher* dose with a meal is reasonable, since this will at least ensure that an effective concentration will eventually be achieved.

All these meal-related troubles have provided a marketing boost to both Cialis (tadalafil) and Stendra (avanafil), neither of which is affected by meals. It's not clear why fatty meals slows the absorption of some PDE5 inhibitors and not others. In the case of Cialis, it may have to do with the fact that it reaches peak concentration later than its two competitors (at about two hours after absorption rather than one hour) so that the meal effect just doesn't have a chance to show up. This is purely conjecture on my part, however, and the logic clearly would not apply to Stendra, which has a more rapid onset than any of its competitors.

Drug-Drug Interactions and Absorption

While most drug-drug interactions relate to biotransformation (see Chapter 6), some are actually a function of interactions in *absorption*. The most common culprits are the opiate narcotics, including codeine, Percocet (acetaminophen & oxycodone), Vicodin (hydrocodone & acetaminophen), and OxyContin (oxycodone). Patients on these meds might require higher doses of certain psych meds to achieve therapeutic levels. While these interactions are real, exactly how they affect the doses you should prescribe have not yet been worked out, and there is likely much inter-individual variation.

The Special Case of Grapefruit

The lowly grapefruit can cause quite a bit of mischief for patients. It increases the concentrations of certain drugs, though the mechanism has nothing to do with absorption. Instead, it affects biotransformation. Grapefruit inhibits the CYP3A enzyme system (which we cover in more detail in Chapter 6), and therefore can increase concentrations of several drugs, including some hypnotics, BuSpar (buspirone), methadone,

Tegretol (carbamazepine), tricyclics, Seroquel (quetiapine), and PDE5 inhibitors. (See the table in the Appendix, Psychiatric Drug Interactions by Enzyme Family.)

Important Drug/Food Interactions in Psychiatric Practice

Medication	Interaction	Instructions
Venlafaxine XR, buspirone	Food eases GI distress	Take with food
Lithium, divalproex	Food eases GI distress	Take with food
Sildenafil, vardenafil	Food delays and decreases absorption by 1 hour	Wait 1 hour after meal
Zolpidem, zaleplon	Food delays and decreases absorption	Wait 1 hour after meal
Ziprasidone, lurasidone	Food increases absorption by 2- to 3-fold	Take with food
Sertraline	Food increases absorption, Cmax by 25%	Take with food
Vilazodone	Food increases absorption by 50%	Take with food
Psychostimulants	Variable, may delay absorption, often decreases appetite	Take after meal to prevent weight loss

Sources: Physician's Desk Reference; Food Medication Interactions, 13th Ed. (see bibliography for details).
Christina Won, Food-drug interactions in Psychiatry: What Clinicians need to know. June 19, 2014, *Psychiatric Times* http://bit.ly/10A2vxo

NOTE: I didn't include MAOI-tyramine interactions in the table because these are covered in detail in Chapter 8.

Chapter 3

Half-Life, Onset, Duration: Some Concepts to Help You Prescribe

The half-life is the time required for half of a drug to leave your patient's body. Five is the magic number: it takes five half-lives for a drug to reach a steady state, at which point you can order a blood level that is fairly reliable. And it also takes five half-lives for the drug to be completely out of the patient's system after stopping it.

In order to be a great psychopharmacologist, you really have to commit certain half-lives to memory, because you will be using this information constantly in making dosing decisions. So I've created a half-life table for you to memorize (on next page and also reproduced in the appendix). The numbers aren't strictly accurate, but they're close enough. I rounded up or down liberally in order to make these easier to memorize.

There's also a column listing the approximate times required for each drug to reach steady state or elimination from the body. Of course, you can always simply multiply half-life by five to figure this out for yourself, but the table is a useful quick reference for those of us who don't want to have to think any more than we need to. In order to understand what steady state actually means, read the relevant section below.

A Brief Lesson in Pharmacokinetics

Let's look at some standard concepts in pharmacokinetics that will help us to predict how quickly a given drug will reach a therapeutic serum level.

Half-Lives of Psychiatric Medications

Medication	Half-life (in hours, except where indicated)	Time to Steady State or Elimination
Anti-anxiety		
BuSpar	2 hours	10 hours
Ativan, Xanax	10 hours	2 days
Klonopin, Valium	40 hours	8 days
Sleeping Pills		
Sonata	1 hour	5 hours
Ambien	2.5 hours	12 hours
Lunesta	6 hours	30 hours
Restoril, Trazodone	10 hours	2 days
Antidepressants		
Effexor	6 hours	30 hours
Parnate	2.5 hours	12 hours
Cymbalta, Fetzima (levomilnacipran), Nardil, Pristiq	12 hours	3 days
Celexa, Clomipramine, Desipramine, EMSAM, Lexapro, Paxil, Remeron, Wellbutrin, Viibryd, Zoloft	24 hours	5 days
Nortriptyline	36 hours	8 days
Vortioxetine (Brintellix)	3 days	15 days
Prozac	10–14 days	50 days
Mood Stabilizers		
Depakote	10 hours	2 days
Tegretol	24 hours initially, then 15 hours after auto-induction	3 days
Lithium, Lamictal	24 hours	5 days

Continued on next page

Half-Lives of Psychiatric Medications
(continued)

Medication	Half-life (in hours, except where indicated)	Time to Steady State or Elimination
Antipsychotics		
Seroquel, Geodon	6 hours	30 hours
Clozaril, Trilafon	10 hours	2 days
Fanapt, Haldol, Invega, Latuda, Risperdal, Saphris, Zyprexa	24 hours	5 days
Abilify	3 days	15 days
PDE5 Inhibitors		
Levitra, Stendra (avanafil), Viagra	4 hours	1 day
Cialis	18 hours	4 days

Note: Half-life figures derive from a variety of sources, including drug package inserts, textbooks, and online databases. These figures are all *approximate*, and wide variations in half-life estimates are often published, depending on the pharmacokinetic studies referenced.

After a patient ingests a drug, it gets absorbed and fairly quickly reaches a peak concentration, termed "Cmax." The time required for a particular drug to reach Cmax is called its "Tmax." Note that Tmax is not the same thing as onset of effect. For example, Viagra takes about an hour (without food) to reach Cmax, but its onset of action is 20 to 30 minutes. This is because most drugs start to affect the body at concentrations lower than their maximum eventual concentrations. For Viagra (and this is true for benzodiazepines as well), the effective concentration is attained well before Cmax.

After Cmax, the concentration comes gradually down, eventually reaching a "Cmin," or "trough concentration," just before the next dose is taken. Graphically, the best way to comprehend these concepts is to look at a "concentration-time curve," as printed in the *Physicians' Desk Reference* (PDR) for most drugs. It shows how the amount of a single dose of a drug in the blood varies over time.

Concentration-Time Curve

If you bother to read much of the promotional literature for extended-release drugs, you'll likely see lots of curves like this and you'll read about "AUC," meaning "area under the curve." The

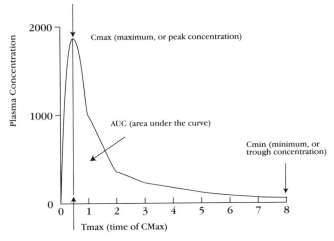

AUC is a measure of the total amount of drug absorbed by the body, and the extended-release promos use the term to prove that a once-a-day ER formulation leads to an AUC comparable to BID or TID dosing of the IR formulation. We'll scrutinize the value of ER compounds more closely in Chapter 4.

How Lithium Reaches Steady State in Five Half-Lives

Have you ever wondered what steady state actually means, why it takes five half-lives to achieve it, and what makes it the right time to get an accurate blood level? The answer is not as simple as you might think. A common misconception about steady state is that it means that the serum drug levels are the same throughout the day. Not true. Steady state means that your body is eliminating the drug at the same overall rate as you are ingesting it.

To understand how this works, let's look at the example of starting a patient on lithium, a drug that requires periodic drug monitoring to ensure an adequate dose and to prevent toxicity. The half-life of lithium is about 24 hours. Let's assume we start our patient on 600 mg QD on Day 1 (see "Day 1 Max" in the chart below). Twenty-four hours later, just before his second dose on Day 2, the amount left in his body is 300 mg ("Day 2 Min"), because 24 hours (one half-life) have passed, and therefore the patient has excreted half of the initial amount. He then swallows another 600 mg for his Day 2 dose, resulting in a Day 2 Max of 600 mg + 300 mg = 900 mg. On Day 3, he starts the day with half of 900 mg, or 450 mg, and after his 600 mg dose he has 1050 mg. And so on. As you can see, with each passing day, the blood levels—both peak and trough—become more and more

Body Content of Lithium in Milligrams	Day 1	Day 2		Day 3		Day 4	
	Max	Min	Max	Min	Max	Min	Max
	600	300	900	450	1050	525	1125
	Day 5		Day 6		Day 7		
	Min	Max	Min	Max	Min	Max	
	562	1162	581	1181	590	1190	

predictable. They still fluctuate by 600 mg a day, but the peak and trough are relatively stable.

And this explains why we wait five half-lives before drawing a blood level. At Day 2, the trough blood level would be 300, and at Day 3, it would be 450. There's a big difference between 300 mg and 450 mg, which shows why drawing blood levels too early yields unreliable results. However, a blood level draw at Day 5 (562) is not much different from Day 7 (590), which in turn will not be much different from the result on Day 300, as long as the dose stays at 600 mg. Eventually, a limit is reached, with the peak hovering around 1200 and the trough around 600.

Understanding Half-Life Helps You to Know When to Get a Blood Level

So when is it helpful to know about the concept of steady state? Mainly when you are trying to figure out the right time to get a blood level on a patient taking lithium, Depakote (sodium divalproex), or Tegretol. If you get a level too early (before five half-lives), your trough level will underestimate the actual blood level after steady state is achieved.

By the way, there's a strange myth floating around that drugs with long half-lives take longer to "work" than drugs with short half-lives. Apparently this is a result of a misinterpretation of the meaning of steady state. True, long half-life meds take longer to get to steady state. Prozac (fluoxetine), in concert with its norfluoxetine metabolite, for example, with a half-life of about two weeks, takes 2 ½ months to reach steady state. Nonetheless, Prozac works just as quickly as short half-life antidepressants (Gelenberg AJ & Chesen CL, *J Clin Psychiatry* 2000;61(10):712–721). Evidently, serotonin receptors aren't waiting around until Prozac reaches steady state.

Understanding Half-Life Helps You to Optimize Duration of Action

In order to optimize the duration of action, we have to dose our medications just right, and a medication's half-life is our most important dosing guide. We dose a short half-life medication more frequently than a long half-life medication. This much is clear. However, exactly how we should use the half-life to make our dosing decisions can get confusing. The oft-cited guideline that the dosage interval should be equivalent to the half-life is completely inapplicable at times.

For example, Xanax (alprazolam), the poster child of anxiolytics requiring frequent dosing, is generally prescribed in every four to six hour increments. However, the half-life of Xanax is not six hours, but 10 to 12 hours. This means that after six hours, fully 75% of the initial Xanax dose is still coursing through your patient's bloodstream. And yet, when it comes to benzos, anxious patients are very sensitive to even tiny changes in blood levels, and when 25% of the drug is gone, they feel the need for the next dose. Similarly, Klonopin has a long half-life of 30 to 40 hours, implying that once a day dosing would work just fine. But flesh-and-blood patients say that they need it on a BID or even TID schedule.

How do extended-release versions of medications increase duration of action? *Not* by increasing the half-life, which is an inherent biochemical property of a given drug that doesn't vary. Rather, ER drugs work by controlling the release of drug from the tablet, so that absorption is stretched way out. For example, Xanax XR (extended-release), is Xanax packaged in a kind of pill that controls the release of Xanax and maintains it at a constant blood level for about twice as long as immediate-release Xanax. This formulation effectively turns it into a pharmacokinetic duplicate of Klonopin.

Another way to increase a drug's duration of action is by simply increasing the dose, a psychopharmacologic maneuver that doesn't sound like it should work, at least not at first glance. After all, the half-life doesn't change no matter what the dose, so why should simply giving *more* of a drug increase duration of action?

We'll explain this with the example of using Ritalin (methylphenidate) to treat a child with ADHD. Let's assume that the 20 mg QD that you have been prescribing is not quite getting him through the half-day of summer school he has to attend. You consider switching him to a longer-acting formulation, but his parents are concerned about over-exposure to stimulants, especially since he has already been losing weight on Ritalin. Knowing about the principles of pharmacokinetics, you suggest slightly *increasing* the Ritalin as a solution.

Why should this work?

Ritalin has a half-life of about two hours. Now, let's say that the minimum effective concentration of Ritalin in the blood stream is 1 "unit"/ml, and that 20 mg QD produces a blood level of 4 units/ml soon after your patient swallows the pill (I use the term "unit" for ease of explanation—the actual blood concentration will vary from patient to patient). Two hours later, the concentration has decreased by 50%, to 2 units/ml, and two hours after that, it has fallen to 1 unit/ml. Thus, a total of four hours after ingestion, the blood concentration of Ritalin has fallen just below the efficacy threshold—which is just another way of saying that its duration of action is four hours.

Let's say you want to eke out just one more hour of effectiveness. If you increased the Ritalin dose from 20 mg to 30 mg QD, this would increase the initial concentration from 4 units/ml to 6 units/ml. Two half-lives (four hours) later, the blood level would be 1.5 units/ml, above the therapeutic threshold, and you still have another hour of drug action ahead of you. Presto! You've used your superior knowledge of pharmacokinetics to avoid the hassles of a formulation change.

Of course, this trick has its limits, mainly involving side effects that you may cause by dumping such a high dose into your patient's body all at once. In such cases, it's better to use an ER version of Ritalin.

Understanding Half-Life Helps You to Avoid Withdrawal Symptoms–Sort of

In the world of antidepressants, the half-life helps us understand which drugs are more likely to lead to discontinuation side effects. For example, Effexor (venlafaxine), with its half-life of only six hours, often causes dizziness, nausea, and anxiety upon stopping it, whereas Prozac, with its forever half-life of five days (more than two weeks or so if you count its active metabolite), almost never causes withdrawal symptoms.

However, the half-life rule doesn't always help us. For example, Paxil (paroxetine) arguably leads the pack in withdrawal risk, causing problems in at least 60% of patients who stop it (Rosenbaum JF et al, *Biol Psychiatry* 1998;44(2):77–87). But its half-life of 24 hours is no shorter than those of Zoloft, Celexa (citalopram), and Lexapro (escitalopram). What gives?

The Paxil story may have to do with how it is metabolized. As you'll learn in Chapter 6, Paxil is metabolized primarily by the P450 2D6 enzyme. But it also inhibits the action of this enzyme, meaning that Paxil inhibits its own metabolism. When you stop taking Paxil, its concentration gradually decreases according to its 24 hour half-life. But as it begins to leave the body, the 2D6 enzymes that it was inhibiting start to rev back up, accelerating Paxil's degradation. This speeded-up disappearance may be what causes the high rate of Paxil withdrawal symptoms (Fava GA & Grandi S, *J Clin Psychopharmacol* 1995;15(5):374–375).

Another drug that doesn't fit neatly into the half-life theory of withdrawal is Serzone (nefazodone), which, with a half-life of six hours, should cause raging discontinuation symptoms. Its lower risk might be related to the fact that it isn't an SSRI. While Serzone does inhibit serotonin reuptake, it also blocks Serotonin Type 2 receptors, and this might prevent withdrawal problems.

What Understanding Half-Life Doesn't Help You With

What does half-life have to do with the fabled and mysterious delay in antidepressant effect? Probably nothing at all. To begin with, the very notion that antidepressants take a month to work has been largely debunked. An article by Posternak and Zimmerman at Brown University (*J Clin Psychiatry* 2005;66(2):148–158) described a meta-analysis of antidepressant trials, and concluded that 60% of improvement on ADs occurs within the first two weeks.

But even acknowledging that there is a delay in antidepressant response, the reason for this has nothing to do with time to reach steady state, since many other meds we prescribe manage to work on the brain immediately, including Klonopin, whose half-life, at 40 hours, is longer than all ADs except Prozac. The antidepressant delay is all about the pharmacodynamics of these meds, including receptor effects, G-proteins, alterations in transcription, and other complicated stuff that you'll find in Steven Stahl's textbook, *Essential Psychopharmacology: Neuroscientific Basis and Practical Applications*. (Remember that pharmacodynamics is the effect of the drug on the body, while pharmacokinetics is the effect of the body on the drug.)

Discussing Half-Lives with Your Patients: A Clinical Anecdote

Aside from allowing you to get fancy with your dosing, knowing a lot about half-lives helps you to explain things to your patients, which, in my experience, increases adherence to medication regimens.

For example, I once switched a patient from Xanax 1 mg TID to Klonopin. I wrote enough Klonopin for him to take 1 mg TID if need be, just to make extra certain that he wouldn't go into benzodiazepine withdrawal. But I also told him that he would eventually be able to get by with 1 mg BID. He was very skeptical, since he was hooked on the idea of taking that midday dose of something to prevent panic. I explained to him that, since the half-life of Klonopin is 40 hours, in the 12 hours between BID dosing, only about ¼ of 50%, or about 12%, of his Klonopin would be metabolized. "At the end of the day, you still have almost 90% of the original amount of Klonopin in your bloodstream." This made sense to him, and he was quickly able to wean himself down to Klonopin 1 mg BID.

"Linear" vs. "Non-Linear" Pharmacokinetics

These somewhat confusing terms are not commonly relevant in psychiatry, thankfully enough. Almost all psychiatric drugs exhibit linear pharmacokinetics, which means that the serum level of drug in the bloodstream is directly proportional to the dose. This means that if your patient doubles her dose, her serum level doubles as well. Thus, the common practice of gradually titrating the dose of a drug upward until there is a clinical effect is appropriate in most cases.

Several drugs used in psychiatry have *non-linear pharmacokinetics:* Prozac, Paxil, fluvoxamine, BuSpar, Tegretol, Depakene, and Neurontin (gabapentin) (Schwab M et al, Eds. *Pharmacogenomics in Psychiatry.* Basel, Switzerland: Karger; 2010). This means that as you increase the dose of these medications, the serum levels may increase more or less than would be predicted by a straight line on a graph. The reasons vary by the drug. Some drugs, like Paxil, inhibit their own metabolism, so their concentrations tend to rise faster than predicted. Other drugs, like Tegretol, induce their own metabolism, causing concentrations to increase more slowly. In clinical practice, non-linearity of pharmacokinetics is primarily an issue when using those that are particularly toxic at high serum levels (such as Tegretol and Depakene), especially in patients with impaired hepatic functioning.

Potency vs. Effectiveness

The term "potency" often causes confusion for our patients, and occasionally for clinicians as well. In general, potency refers to a drug's power per unit, or the amount of pharmacological activity per milligram. This issue sometimes comes up when we switch from one medication to another. For example, switching from 20 mg of Prozac to 150 mg of Effexor XR sometimes causes patients to wonder if we are trying to overdose them. Conversely (and probably more relevant to patient safety), when we switch from, say, 100 mg of Zoloft to 20 mg of Celexa, some patients may think that they are being underdosed and may then increase their doses between visits if they do not see a rapid improvement. Clarifying the difference between potency and dose can head off such a problem.

Chapter 4

Tweaking Pills:
How Extended-Release
Medications Work

These days, you can't really show your face as a self-respecting pharmaceutical executive if you haven't launched at least one "extended-release" product within the past year. We are increasingly bombarded by "SR" (slow-release), "CR" (continuous-release), "ER" (extended-release), or "XR" ("Xtended"-release) versions of drugs. They obviously have certain advantages, but we psychiatrists have probably been excessively gullible in terms of swallowing (so to speak) the drugmakers' claims that we should be switching over to these products. In this chapter we'll take a closer look at the most popular ER products and decide which ones are great, and which ones should be used with a good dose of caution.

In the old days, you prescribed a simple pill or capsule that would begin to disintegrate in the stomach, releasing all of the drug pretty quickly. The drug's serum concentration would spike up quickly, and then come back down, leading to pretty low "trough" levels before the next dose.

So, what's the problem with fluctuating concentrations of drugs? One problem is a bad side effect profile, caused by a higher-than-necessary peak concentration soon after your patient takes the drug. Another, opposite problem is inadequate efficacy during the period when the concentration is at its *lowest* level. This efficacy issue is particularly problematic for anti-seizure meds, cardiac meds, and antibiotics. In each of these cases, inadequate blood levels can lead to catastrophic medical consequences.

Are Consistent Drug Levels Important in Psychiatry?

In psychiatry, consistent blood levels appear to be important for relatively few situations, such as the use of benzodiazepines for panic disorder, stimulants for ADHD, and lithium for preventing mania. With benzodiazepines, for example, repeated periods of low drug concentration throughout the day lead to the "clock watching" that patients on immediate-release Xanax are famous for. This is why longer-acting Klonopin (clonazepam) quickly became so popular, and why Xanax XR was released, in an effort to grab some market share away from Klonopin.

But in the world of antidepressants and antipsychotics, smoothing out fluctuating drug levels doesn't necessarily lead to better efficacy. We know, for example, that the two major extended-release antidepressants, Effexor XR and Paxil CR, are no more effective than their short-acting immediate-release cousins. We also know that for another short half-life antidepressant, Serzone, single dosing at night appears to work just as well as twice daily dosing, and with less daytime sedation (Voris JC et al, *Pharmacotherapy* 1998;18(2):379–380).

Of the newer antipsychotics, the package insert recommends twice daily dosing for Geodon and Seroquel, both of which have half-lives of about six hours. However, one double-blind study of 21 hospitalized patients showed no difference in response to Seroquel whether it was dosed once at bedtime or twice daily (Chengappa KNR et al, *Can J Psychiatry* 2003;48(3):187–194). In general, then, there is no compelling efficacy argument for ensuring that blood levels of antidepressants or antipsychotics stay consistent throughout the day.

Tolerability, however, is another story. Formulations that smooth out the peaks *do* seem to reduce the side effect burden, the most spectacular example of which is Effexor XR. Some of you may recall that when Effexor was first introduced in 1995 it was nicknamed "side effexor," because of a harsh combination of nausea, daytime sedation, and nighttime insomnia. In 1998, Effexor XR was introduced, and was tolerated so much better that it became one of the most widely prescribed antidepressants. This improved tolerability theme will repeat itself in many of the examples of specific ER formulations examined below.

With regard to antipsychotics, there is one study comparing Seroquel XR with generic quetiapine IR. Conducted by AstraZeneca, it involved randomly assigning healthy subjects to one of the two versions, then measuring levels of sedation at different time points. Quetiapine IR caused more sedation after one hour than Seroquel XR, but there was no difference between the two at seven hours or 14 hours post-dose (Datto C et al, *Clin Ther* 2009;31(3):492–502). This study is not exactly a ringing endorsement of XR, because we often choose quetiapine over other antipsychotics precisely because it can do double duty as a sleeping pill. If the XR version lacks this effect, it's less useful overall.

The Wellbutrin Story: Which Version to Choose

With three versions of Wellbutrin (bupropion) on the market, it's important to review each one's relative benefits (or lack thereof).

What are the differences among these formulations? All three versions contain the same molecule, of course (bupropion), and there is no difference in antidepressant efficacy among them. The table on the next page compares the three versions on pharmacokinetic parameters, and you can see that there is a major difference between IR and the other two versions.

As you might predict, the immediate-release Wellbutrin reaches its Cmax (maximum concentration) much sooner than the others, and reaches a higher concentration. If you were to look at the concentration-time curve, Wellbutrin IR has a saw tooth pattern, with three Grand Teton-type peaks corresponding to TID dosing; SR has two gentler peaks; and XL has only one Appalachian appearing peak (see Figure 1 on next page).

Wellbutrin Comparison

	Bupropion IR (100 mg TID)	Buproprion SR (150 mg BID)	Wellbutrin XL (300 mg QAM)
Tmax	1.5 hours	2.5 hours	5 hours
Steady state Cmax (ng/ml)	144	112	119
Steady state Cmin (ng/ml)	30	26	23
Price (1 mo. supply)	$24 (generic)	$44 (generic)	$56 (brand)

Source for prices: Boston area CVS pharmacies, December 2014

Figure 1:

Steady State Plasma Level Concentrations for
Wellbutrin 300 mg/day for IR, SR, and XL Formulations

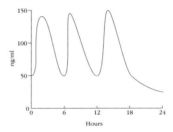

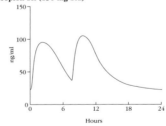

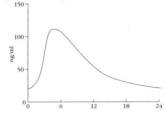

Source: Data from GlaxoSmithKline, Research Triangle Park, NC

Abbreviations: IR = immediate-release, SR = sustained-release, XL = extended-release

So What Do These Different Profiles Imply for Us Clinicians?

Regarding convenience, once daily dosing is certainly more convenient than the BID or TID dosing recommended for other Wellbutrin formulations. The Wellbutrin SR package insert recommends taking no more than 200 mg at a time, but there are no data indicating that taking 300 mg at once is hazardous, and clearly many patients do just that. There is also no evidence that smoothing out the fluctuations in Wellbutrin blood levels makes the drug a more effective antidepressant. When Wellbutrin XL was first introduced, the manufacturer's promotional material emphasized that the serum level of bupropion is lower at bedtime in patients taking Wellbutrin XL 300 mg QAM than in patients taking Wellbutrin SR 150 mg BID. The implication was that XL may cause less insomnia than SR, but thus far there is no clinical data demonstrating that this is true.

Wellbutrin and the Risk of Seizure

With Wellbutrin, the main side effect that we worry about is seizure. Wellbutrin's package insert is clear, recommending that in order to decrease the risk of seizure, the total dose should be no more than 450 mg QD, and that (for the IR and SR versions) no single dose should be more than 150 mg for IR or 200 mg for SR. If you look closely at the studies, you find that the seizure rate for doses 300 mg or below is 0.1%, about the same as any antidepressant (Fava M et al, *Prim Care Companion J Clin Psychiatry* 2005;7(3):106–113). This increases fourfold, to 0.4%, among patients taking 450 mg QD. Going up to 600 mg QD increases the seizure risk substantially, to about 3%. It's important to realize that all of these data were derived from studies of the immediate and sustained-release versions. There are no seizure data available for the new XL form, but, according to the company, the numbers are likely to be similar ("Incidence of Seizure Reported with Wellbutrin XL," monograph available from GlaxoSmithKline).

So the bottom line is that the lower the dose of Wellbutrin, the lower the seizure risk, regardless of the formulation.

The Paxil CR Story: A Little Less Nausea

In 2002, GlaxoSmithKline (GSK) had a problem: Paxil was about to go off patent. It soon launched Paxil CR, which is different from Paxil in two ways. First, it is enteric coated, preventing it from dissolving in the stomach. This is a good thing, because it decreases the percentage of patients with week-one nausea from 23% with Paxil IR to 14% with Paxil CR. However, by week two, there are no significant differences in nausea rates between the formulations (Golden R et al, *J Clin Psychiatry* 2002;63(7):577–584).

The second difference is the "geomatrix" interior, which allows Paxil to be released gradually over several hours. This feature in itself appears to yield little benefit, although theoretically those rare patients who experience Paxil withdrawal between daily doses might see these symptoms disappear with the CR version.

Incidentally, fancy new formulations can sometimes bring their own special problems, as GSK discovered in 2005 when the FDA ordered its Puerto Rican production facility to temporarily stop making Paxil CR. Apparently, pharmacists had noticed that some batches of the medication were defective. These pills tended to come apart while they were in the bottle in such a way that all the active paroxetine ended up on one side and the extended-release fillers ended up on the other (Harris G. FDA Seizes Millions of Pills From Pharmaceutical Plants. *New York Times.* March 5, 2005). Eventually, they fixed the problem and were allowed to rev up their factory once again.

The Lithium Story:
For the Kidneys, Less May Be More

The lithium story is very much like the Wellbutrin story in terms of formulations, but the rationale for going "fancy" is less compelling for lithium. As shown on the next page, there are three different formulations of lithium: the original immediate-release lithium carbonate, the extended-release "Lithobid," and the even further extended-release "Eskalith CR." All three versions are available as generics, and this is reflected in the pricing listed in the chart below.

	Lithium Carbonate (300 mg TID)	Lithobid (900 mg split BID)	Eskalith CR (450 mg BID)
Tmax	2 hours	4 hours	4 hours
Price (1 mo. supply of generic versions)	$9	$17	$17

Source for prices: Boston area CVS pharmacies, September 2014

There is no demonstrated efficacy advantage for patients taking longer-acting versions of lithium, although patients tend to report fewer GI side effects with the ER formulations. However, there is evidence that taking regular lithium (lithium carbonate) *once* a day leads to fewer problems with polyuria than taking it *twice* a day, probably because it exposes the kidneys to lithium for a relatively short period of time (Gitlin M, *Drug Saf* 1999;20(3):231–243). The implication is that we should avoid the longer-acting versions of lithium if at all possible, in the interest of being kind to our patients' kidneys. A prudent beginning dosing strategy is to start with good old lithium carbonate, and dose it all in the evening.

The Depakote Story: ER Better Tolerated, but Less Effective?

Like lithium, the Depakote story is one of initial enthusiasm for the ER version, which has been somewhat tempered by recent data.

To begin with, let's try to bring some clarity to the multiple confusing names for Depakote. The basic, irreducible molecule here is valproic acid, also known as valproate, and the brand name of this is "Depakene," not Depakote.

Depakote is known generically as "sodium divalproex," and is formed by adding sodium hydroxide to two valproic acid molecules, yielding a molecule that is double the size of Depakene, but which gets broken right back down to humble valproic acid in the stomach.

The "kote" in Depakote refers to the fact that it comes in an enteric-coated tablet. It tends to cause fewer GI side effects than Depakene, is absorbed more slowly, and has a somewhat longer half-life (12 hours vs. eight hours). Because of this, you will sometimes hear Depakote described as a "delayed-release" version of valproic acid (and I will use "Depakote DR" to distinguish it from Depakote ER).

Depakote ER is an extended-release version of Depakote DR and is FDA-approved for once daily dosing. Of course, most of us have become accustomed to dosing regular Depakote DR all at night, so the Depakote ER convenience advantage is pretty much a non-issue. The real issues here are both efficacy and side effects— does Depakote ER beat its less fancy cousin on either measure?

For efficacy, the answer is probably no, according to a 2007 study in which 21 patients with bipolar disorder switched from one formulation to the other. There were no differences in efficacy or tolerability between Depakote DR and Depakote ER, even when Depakote DR was dosed once a day as opposed to its approved twice a day dosing. However, the study did provide the clinical pearl which is that if you switch patients from Depakote DR to Depakote ER, you need to increase the dose by about 20% to maintain the same serum levels.

However, a larger study funded by Abbott (the manufacturer of Depakote ER), reported that patients who were switched from Depakote DR to Depakote ER reported a reduction of tremor, weight gain, and GI problems on the newer formulation (Smith MC et al, *Epilepsy Behav* 2004;5(5):746–751). This was an open label trial, meaning that both the patients and researchers knew who was receiving the "new and improved agent," leading to the possibility of reporting bias; but if this finding is generalizable, it would be a fairly strong argument to start most patients on Depakote ER for tolerability reasons alone.

However, Depakote in general may be less effective than its cousin Depakene (valproic acid). In a study of 9,260 patients admitted to inpatients psychiatric units, patients who were started on

Depakote had a 33% longer hospital stay than patients started on standard valproic acid (Wassef AA et al, *Am J Psychiatry* 2005;162(2):330–339). While Depakote was tolerated somewhat better, its use was associated with lower valproic acid levels, which was probably why it was less effective. Thus, it appears that if you are treating an acutely ill patient, you should consider starting with the short-acting valproic acid in order to get rapid efficacy, and then switch over to Depakote (either regular or ER) if tolerability becomes an issue.

Psychostimulants: A Pharmacokinetic Primer

For an extended-release enthusiast, the world of psychostimulants is like Jerusalem. It's where extended-release formulations all began, and where they return year after year. Both Ritalin SR and Dexedrine Spansules have been in existence since the 1960s, and over time, other ER products such as Concerta, Ritalin LA, and Adderall XR have joined the fray. There are at least 18 FDA-approved psychostimulant formulations...and counting (see table on next page).

There are two basic types of stimulants: methylphenidate (Ritalin and its knock-offs) and amphetamine (Dexedrine and Adderall). Within each of these large categories, there are subcategories, depending on the pharmacokinetics of the specific drug. The three typical subcategories are: (1) Short-acting—3 to 5 hours; (2) Intermediate-acting—5 to 8 hours; (3) Long-acting—8 to 12 hours. Of course, it gets more complicated than this, because within the intermediate and long-acting groups, you have meds that release the stimulant *continuously,* and others that release it in stages, often mimicking the action of taking an immediate-release stimulant twice a day.

We'll begin with the **methylphenidate** preparations. There are three immediate-release (IR) players: **Ritalin, Focalin,** and **Methylin. Ritalin and Methylin are identical,** in that both are 50:50 mixtures of d- and l-methylphenidate. Focalin is purified d-methylphenidate. The

Short-Acting
Dexedrine
Focalin
Methylin CT
Methylin Oral Solution
Ritalin

Intermediate-Acting
Adderall
Metadate ER
Ritalin SR

Long-Acting
Adderall XR
Concerta
Daytrana
Dexedrine SR
Focalin XR
Metadate CD
Quillivant XR
Ritalin LA
Vyvanse

idea here is that since the d-isomer of methylphenidate is the more biologically active one, getting rid of the l-isomer might improve matters by reducing side effects (though there is as yet no evidence that this is true) and by making it more potent. (True, it is more potent, in that 10 mg of Focalin = 20 mg of Ritalin, but this presents no obvious clinical advantage.)

For kids who hate swallowing pills, there are now three methylphenidate options: **Methylin CT** (chewable tablet), **Methylin Oral Solution,** and **Daytrana,** the methylphenidate patch, which is officially known as **the methylphenidate transdermal system,** or **MTS.**

Ritalin SR is intermediate-acting, and is one of the oldest sustained-release drugs around. It's basically just methylphenidate packed in wax, which substantially delays its absorption. Thus, whereas the peak absorption of Ritalin IR occurs about *two hours* after ingestion, the peak absorption of Ritalin SR occurs about *four to five hours* after ingestion.

There are five long-acting versions of methylphenidate. **Ritalin LA** is a capsule filled with beads. Half the beads are immediate-release methylphenidate, and the other half are enteric-coated, delayed-release beads. Giving 20 mg of Ritalin LA is like giving two 10 mg doses of regular Ritalin about four hours apart. **Metadate CD** is just like Ritalin LA, a capsule filled with immediate- and delayed-release methyl-phenidate beads. The difference is that only 30% of the beads are immediate-release, and 70% are delayed-release. So if your patient needs more of a stimulant punch later in the day, Metadate CD might be just the ticket. **Focalin XR** contains roughly the same combination of immediate- and delayed-release beads as Ritalin LA, but it is all purified *d*-methylphenidate.

Concerta has the most interesting delivery system of them all. It looks like a regular tablet, but within it are three compartments: two layers of methylphenidate, and one "push" layer with an osmotically active polymer. Surrounding the whole thing is a methylphenidate overcoat, which dissolves rapidly, delivering 22% of the dose within the first hour. Then, water seeps in through a semipermeable membrane, gradually expanding the polymer compartment, causing drug to slowly escape through a precision drilled orifice at the other end of the tablet. The result? Twelve or so hours of continuously-released methylphenidate.

Finally, Pfizer recently accomplished the neat trick of creating a long-acting liquid version of methylphenidate, called **Quillivant XR.** It lasts eight to 12 hours, and is the right choice for those pill-o-phobes in your practice who need all day coverage.

Now for the amphetamine preparations. **Dexedrine** is an immediate-release preparation of d-amphetamine. **Dexedrine Spansules** are classified as long-acting, and are bead-filled capsules (50% IR and 50% SR) that provide an initial dose of amphetamine, followed by continuously releasing drug, with a peak plasma level eight hours after ingestion.

The immediate-release version of **Adderall** lasts somewhat longer than any of the IR versions of any of the other stimulants, meaning that Adderall can sometimes be dosed once a day. There is also an **Adderall XR,** a capsule with both IR beads (50%) and delayed-release beads (50%). Serum levels peak at seven hours post-ingestion (vs. 3 hours for Adderall IR). And finally, there's **Vyvanse** (lisdexamfetamine), which is basically Dexedrine bound to a lysine molecule. The lysine prevents the drug from becoming active, and can only be cleaved off once Vyvanse is swallowed.

This interesting formulation accomplishes two things: first, it slows down the drug's release, and second, it makes it impossible to abuse by snorting—though it can still be abused by swallowing.

A Patch for ADHD: Daytrana

I mentioned Daytrana, the methylphenidate transdermal system, in passing, but let's return to it, since it is a novel stimulant delivery system. Daytrana consists of methylphenidate molecules mixed in with a couple of different adhesives. When applied to the skin (Novartis recommends that it be applied to the hip), it gradually releases methylphenidate into the bloodstream. How long does it last? It lasts pretty much as long as you wear it. As you can see from the table below, the initial dose contains 27.5 mg in the adhesive. The delivery rate is 1.1 mg per hour. Thus, if you left the patch on for 24 hours, you would be continuously dosed with methylphenidate over that period. Of course, nobody would want this length of exposure, and Novartis specifies a maximum wear time of nine hours. Why nine hours? Because when they tested a 12-hour wear time, the side effect rate was astronomical: a 61% rate of appetite loss and a 47% rate of insomnia in one study (Pelham WE et al, *J*

Daytrana Dosing and Absorption Parameters

Nominal Dose Delivered (mg) Over 9 Hours	Dosage Rate (mg/hr)	Patch Size (cm²)	Methylphenidate Contents per Patch (mg)
10	1.1	12.5	27.5
15	1.6	18.75	41.3
20	2.2	25	55.0
30	3.3	37.5	82.5
* Nominal *in vivo* delivery rate in pediatric subjects aged 6–12 when applied to the hip, based on a 9-hour wear period.			

Source: Daytrana Package Insert

Am Acad Child Adolesc Psychiatry 2005;44(6):522–529). The nine-hour wear time brings these rates down to those typically seen with oral stimulants: appetite loss, 25%, and insomnia, 13%.

As you review the dosing, you might be struck with the apparently low dosing rate. The starting dose delivers only 1.1 mg/hour, yielding a total exposure of 9.9 mg over the recommended nine hour wear time. The maximum dose provides 29.7 mg of methylphenidate over the course of the day, much lower than maximum doses of oral long-acting formulations, such as Concerta, which can be dosed up to 72 mg/day. The reason these small doses work is that Daytrana allows methylphenidate to be absorbed directly into the bloodstream, avoiding the first pass effect. Thus, the transdermally absorbed methylphenidate does not get subjected to the greedy metabolic machinery of the liver until it has had a chance to be distributed to where it counts—the brain.

So far, so good: Daytrana looks like a good option for kids who don't like pills and who need stimulant coverage throughout the day. Unfortunately, there is one troublesome pharmacokinetic parameter that we haven't yet touched on: the lag time to initial detection of methylphenidate in the blood stream. Daytrana's average lag time is reported in the package insert as *3.1 hours.* Assuming that Johnny's classes begins at 7:30 AM, this means that he will need to slap on the patch at 4:30 AM if he wants to start the school day off right. Compare this with Ritalin LA, which has both immediate- and delayed-release beads. According to the package insert, Ritalin LA's lag time is 30 minutes, and it lasts about as long as Daytrana. Furthermore, if Johnny doesn't like to swallow pills, you can open up the capsule and sprinkle the beads on his cereal.

There is another pharmacokinetic idiosyncracy of Daytrana that you need to be aware of—and which some psychiatrists don't realize. After you remove the Daytrana patch, the drug effect persists for up to five hours due to its drug delivery system. Thus, if patients are experiencing side effects later in the day, removing the patch earlier may solve the problem.

Thus, Daytrana gets high marks on formulation novelty, but the long delay before onset of action may limit its practical value in the real world of patient care.

Chapter 5

Now, Get Rid of It:
Biotransformation

First, let's clarify some terms. **Biotransformation** refers to what happens to drugs in the bloodstream before they leave the body. This usually renders them inactive, but it can in some cases cause them to be even more powerful than the parent compounds. **Excretion** and **elimination** refer to how drugs actually leave the body—the vast majority of the time, this is via the kidneys or the GI tract. Another term for biotransformation is simply **drug metabolism,** but over time "drug metabolism" has taken a broader definition encompassing all the things we discuss in this book, including absorption, distribution, biotransformation, and excretion.

Biotransformation is about how drugs get transformed from full and robust molecular form to smaller or altered molecules that can then travel easily through the kidneys or the intestines. But you should know that some drugs get excreted without being transformed at all. In psychiatry, the most famous of these is lithium in its various guises. Lithium simply gets diffused into the kidneys' tubule system and sent to urine. It is known as a metabolically "inert" drug, although pharmacologically, it is highly active, and it can have quite an effect on the kidney, which I will discuss in Chapter 10.

Almost all of the other drugs that we prescribe, however, undergo various chemical reactions before they can be excreted. There are two primary ways that our bodies alter drugs:

1. Phase I reactions (involving Cytochrome P450 enzymes)
2. Phase II reactions, or conjugation (primarily involving glucuronidation)

Phase I Reactions: The P450 System and Others

The enzymes involved in biotransformation have their offices mostly in liver cells, in the linings of the sinuous interior membranes called the "smooth endoplasmic reticulum." These enzymes have many different names and abbreviations, making some discussions of this topic needlessly confusing. The most official term is "Cytochrome P450 enzymes." This is sometimes truncated to "P450 enzymes," and occasionally you'll see the term "microsomal" enzymes, which means the same thing.

By the way, the name Cytochrome P450 enzymes is actually a bit of researcher's jargon. In research laboratories, these enzymes are examined in artificially-created spheres of cellular tissue called "microsomal vesicles." When these enzymes are placed in such vesicles, they give off a colored pigment, and absorb light at a wavelength of 450 nm. Thus, cyto = microsomal vesicles; chrome = colored; P = pigmented; and 450 = 450 nm wavelength of light.

While I know you didn't buy this book to learn about biochemistry, I couldn't resist inserting some biochemistry in the next couple of paragraphs. The reason is that for years I considered the action of P450 enzymes a "black box" of incomprehensibility, and I eventually decided that I felt uncomfortable knowing nothing about what happens to the drugs that I've prescribed to thousands of people. Now, at least I know something about what happens, and if nothing else, this helps me to read the psychiatric literature more intelligently.

The P450 enzymes specialize in turning lipophilic ("fat loving") drugs into water soluble compounds in a process called **Phase I metabolism.** Next, these altered molecules are joined to another molecule to make them really water soluble. This is called **Phase II metabolism** (see next section).

How do drugs become water soluble? By being transformed into "polar" compounds; that is, compounds that are positively charged on one end and negatively charged on the other. These polar molecules are attracted to water, because water is also polar, and the positive side of the drug is attracted to the negative side of H_2O (or in other cases, the negative side of the drug is attracted to the positive side of H_2O). Our kidneys are set up to *excrete* polar compounds and to *reabsorb* lipophilic compounds. If we couldn't polarize things, it would take us months or years to get rid of them. Unfortunately, we have created an entire chapter devoted to the kidney (Chapter 10) in order to torture you into the "wee" hours of the morning.

It turns out that P450 enzymes catalyze three major chemical reactions: oxidation, reduction, and hydrolysis. The point of these reactions is to turn an uncharged molecule into a positively or negatively charged molecule. Once a molecule has a charge (positive or negative), it is more attracted to water (hydrophilic), less attracted to fat (lipophobic), and exits the body more easily.

Oxidation means taking electrons away from a compound, causing it to have a net positive charge. Confusingly, an oxidative reaction does not necessarily mean adding oxygen to the drug; it just means that the drug is left with fewer electrons. There are several ways to achieve this. Prozac, for example, gets oxidized by losing a methyl group (CH_3) and becoming norfluoxetine. (Norfluoxetine happens to be an example of an active metabolite; it continues to block serotonin reuptake transporters until it is further transformed.) Tricyclics get oxidized by gaining a hydroxyl group (OH). While most psych meds are biotransformed via oxidation, a few are biotransformed by **reduction** (adding electrons by adding a hydrogen atom) and still others are biotransformed by **hydrolysis** (adding H_2O, which causes a molecule to split up into two polar molecules).

Phase II Reactions: Conjugation

Conjugation means combining a drug with another molecule, called the "conjugating agent." These agents do two things to medications: first, they render them pharmacologically inactive, and second, they make them more water soluble than the original drug, making it harder for the intestines or the kidney tubules to reabsorb them back into the circulation. So conjugating a drug is quite simple conceptually—it's like putting a heavy, weighted suit on a basketball player, rendering him ineffective at his sport and causing him to leave the court.

Conjugation is known as "Phase II" because it often occurs after the Phase I reactions, in cases where Phase I does not make the drug sufficiently hydrophilic to get eliminated. By far the most common conjugation reaction is **glucuronidation,** in which glucuronic acid ($C_6H_{10}O_6$) is stuck onto a drug, rendering it water soluble (hydrophilic) and lipid insoluble (lipophobic). Glucuronidation is common partly because glucuronic acid is made out of glucose, which is readily available in the body.

In psychiatry, lots of drugs are metabolized mainly by glucuronidation, including Ativan, Restoril (temazepam), Lamictal (lamotrigine), and Depakote. Here's an example of why that matters: Since both Lamictal and Depakote are metabolized by glucuronidation, there's a drug interaction between them. As it turns out, Depakote latches onto the glucuronidation enzyme more strongly than Lamictal, shoving Lamictal aside, preventing it from being metabolized, and thereby increasing its levels to about double what they are otherwise. Thus, when a patient is on Depakote, you have to start Lamictal at 12.5 mg QD rather than 25 mg QD, and you titrate the dose in smaller increments than usual.

To review the essentials of biotransformation: Your average psychiatric medication gets absorbed through the small intestine, gets distributed by the bloodstream to the liver and then to various organs (especially the brain), and then begins its inexorable journey towards oblivion due to close encounters with various enzymes. These enzymes work hard to turn the drugs into polar (hydrophilic) compounds. This involves a variety of maneuvers, including tearing electrons away from the drug (oxidation), stuffing electrons into the drug (reduction), and ripping the molecules apart by offering them some water (hydrolysis). After this "treatment," some drugs are ready to exit right away, either via the kidney or via the bowel. Others require more persuasion, and so are conjugated, which generally means being superglued to glucuronic acid, a highly water soluble compound that effectively ushers drugs out of the body.

As you can see, our patients' bloodstreams may be pretty crowded with enzymes and medications, so it comes as no surprise that there's a fair amount of jostling and pushing going on there. That's the topic of the next chapter.

Chapter 6

Cutting to the Chase: Clinically Relevant Drug-Drug Interactions in Psychiatry

Before you go to the trouble of reading this chapter, I'd like to ask you the following question: Do you believe that drug-drug interactions (DDIs) are even relevant in psychiatry? Because, at least in academic psychiatry, there has historically been a profound split between those who believe that clinically relevant drug interactions are common and those who believe they are rare.

In 2006, two of the best-known experts on drug metabolism debated this issue in the pages of the journal *Neuropsychopharmacology* (2006;31(8):1594–1613). Lindsay DeVane started this remarkable "point-counterpoint" with an article maintaining that clinically significant drug interactions caused by antidepressants are rare, and that the fear of these interactions may have caused clinicians to be overly cautious in prescribing certain drugs.

His argument included the following points:

- Extensive post-marketing surveillance of fluvoxamine (the first SSRI, and the one that inhibits the most enzymes) has not revealed a great deal of adverse events, other than the well-recognized increases in levels of Clozaril (clozapine), Elixophyllin (theophylline), and Coumadin (warfarin).

- Often, even when an inhibitor *does* increase the concentration of a substrate, there are few, if any, clinical consequences. For instance, fluvoxamine increased concentrations of Xanax by 100% in one study, and yet there was no increased sedation, and some cognitive impairment on only one of several cognitive tests.

- Almost all drugs have parallel metabolic systems, allowing alternative enzymes to take over when a particular enzyme is inhibited.

- The common practice of gradually titrating antidepressants compensates for most potential problems. For example, if an antidepressant is prescribed to a patient taking an inhibitor of its metabolism, the low initial starting dose will lead to a relatively high serum concentration. Because of this artificially high serum level, the patient will presumably respond clinically even at the low starting dose, and the clinician, in turn, will be unlikely to raise the dose up to the "standard" effective dose, and the patient will not be exposed to toxic serum levels.

In their response to DeVane's article, Sheldon Preskorn and Steve Werder argued that DDIs can be quite subtle and can mimic various other clinical presentations (*Neuropsychopharmacology op.cit*). These situations are commonly misinterpreted as having causes other than DDIs. The authors provide the following examples:

- A psychiatrist might conclude that a patient has failed an antidepressant trial, when in fact the "failed trial" could be caused by the introduction of a medication that induces the antidepressant's metabolism, causing serum levels to drop to ineffective levels.

- A patient might become labeled as particularly "sensitive" to side effects, when in fact their side effects might reflect high serum levels due to the co-presence of an inhibiting medication.

- A patient taking a pain medication who requests a higher dose may be called a "drug-seeker" when in fact a drug interaction has caused the narcotic to be less effective.

According to Preskorn, it is entirely possible that such hidden drug interactions occur frequently in clinical practice. Since it is very difficult to prove the existence of very subtle interactions via research, we may not have clear documentation of these dangers. Because of this, these authors argue that it makes sense to take the cautious approach and to assume they might happen.

Who's right? I'll let you decide. In this chapter we'll review the potentially important drug interactions in psychiatry. You can let your own clinical experience help you to decide how clinically relevant they truly are.

The Language of Drug Interactions

First, some terminology. A **substrate** is a drug that is metabolized by a particular enzyme. Thus, for example, tricyclics and beta blockers are both substrates of the P450 2D6 enzyme system, because they are both metabolized by that system.

Inhibition happens when two drugs compete for the same metabolic enzyme. One drug (the inhibitor) binds more tightly to the enzyme than the other drug, and the "**victim**" drug then gets stuck in a game of metabolic musical chairs as it scurries around looking for an enzyme system to break it down. This leads, rather quickly, to higher drug levels than otherwise. To complicate things a bit, some drugs specialize in "*non*-competitive inhibition," which is a shameless act of sabotage in which the aggressor drug may not be a substrate of an enzyme, but binds to it anyway, purely in order to disable it. The results are the same as in competitive inhibition — higher levels of the substrate. By the way, the degree of inhibition is dose-related, meaning that the higher the dose of the inhibitor, the more likely and more significant will be the drug-drug interaction.

Induction happens when the "inducing" drug stimulates the production of extra enzymes. If your patient is taking a medication that is metabolized by those same enzymes, then this medication will be broken down more rapidly than normal, leading to lower-than-predicted levels. Unlike inhibition, induction doesn't kick in right after the patient takes the inducing drug, but takes two to three weeks. Why? Because it takes this long for the liver to produce these extra enzymes.

If a patient *stops* taking an inducer or an inhibitor, there will be a corresponding change in the level of the substrate. This is sometimes called **"reversal of inhibition"** or **"reversal of induction."** An example of reversal of inhibition is the patient on Xanax who stops fluvoxamine, which was inhibiting the breakdown of Xanax and causing higher drug levels. Once he stops the fluvoxamine, the P450 3A4 enzymes start breaking down more Xanax, leading to lower than therapeutic Xanax levels and consequent breakthrough panic.

An example of reversal of induction is the patient on Clozaril who finally quits smoking. Since smoking is a potent inducer of clozapine metabolism, taking smoking away eventually leads to a rise in clozapine levels, with the possible consequence of clozapine toxicity, including such symptoms as sedation, orthostatic hypotension, and constipation. Thus, if you admit a patient on Clozaril to a smoke-free unit, you should gradually decrease the dose by about 10% per day for five days, according to one authority (Demler TL, *US Pharm* 2012;37(11):HS16–HS19).

A **pro-drug** is a drug that has little, if any, therapeutic action by itself. In order to work, it must be broken down to an active metabolite. Anything that inhibits the metabolism of a pro-drug will make it less effective, because it will reduce the serum levels of the active metabolite. The most clinically significant of these pro-drugs for psychiatrists are the pain-relievers Ultram (tramadol) and hydrocodone (present in Vicodin and other formulations). They are both substrates of the P450 2D6 enzyme. Thus, adding any of the drugs listed in the table in the Appendix under "2D6 inhibitors" to either Ultram or Vicodin may cause your patient breakthrough pain.

This chapter focuses on **pharmacokinetic** interactions, and not **pharmacodynamic** interactions. Pharmacokinetic interactions involve drugs bumping up against other drugs and effects on drug levels. In Chapter 8, we'll review some of the important interactions in psychiatry that have nothing to do with pharmacokinetics, including the fabled MAOI interactions. These are pharmacodynamic interactions, because they occur at the level of neurotransmitters and receptor sites.

A Common Sense Approach to Drug Interactions

Given all the possible interactions between drugs, a savvy psychopharmacologist will have to consider three possible scenarios when prescribing any drug.

Scenario 1: You are prescribing one drug, and the patient is taking nothing.

What to do: You may think that you don't have to worry about drug interactions. You may be right—if it's really true that your patient is on no other meds. Make sure of this by asking about non-prescription meds or foods that can be involved in drug interactions. Ask: "Do you take any other meds that are not prescribed by anyone, such as St. John's wort, cold medicines with Sudafed, stomach soothers such as Tums or Maalox? Do you drink grapefruit juice or eat a lot of grapefruits?"

Scenario 2: You're prescribing two or more drugs and the patient is taking nothing.

What to do: Ask about non-prescription agents as above. And scrutinize your choice of drugs to make sure there are no interactions between them—or if there are, adjust the dose accordingly.

Scenario 3: You're prescribing one or more meds to someone who is taking one or more meds.

What to do: You have to consider two directions of potential drug interactions. First, your new drugs may affect the existing drugs, by increasing or decreasing levels. Second, the existing drugs may affect the new drugs. Finally, ask about OTCs and grapefruit.

It's Vicious Out There:
Dealing with Drug-Interaction Information Overload

The amount of information relating to drug interactions is overwhelming. Luckily, there are several web-based charts and software programs that are helpful for quickly looking up interactions.

Dr. David Flockhart's site http://www.drug-interactions.com (make sure to include a dash between "drug" and "interactions" in order to arrive at the correct site) lists a very comprehensive list of drugs categorized by substrates, inducers, and inhibitors. If you click on a specific drug, you'll get linked to a journal article backing up the listed interaction. It's a great site, but it still forces you to do the thinking, unlike the products below in which you simply submit the drug names and get back the interactions.

There are many companies offering to sell or to give you drug interactions software these days. Two free tools include Epocrates' "Interaction Check (Multicheck)" (http://www.epocrates.com, or downloadable to your smartphone as an app) and Medscape's "Drug Interaction Checker" (http://reference.medscape.com/drug-interactionchecker, or smartphone app). They are similar, with user-friendly interfaces allowing you to input as many meds as you'd like to ascertain potential interactions. Epocrates requires that you register to use their tool, whereas Medscape does not. While the price is right, I've found that both are somewhat blunt instruments and tend to report many "significant" interactions, which are not necessarily so. For example, if you type in any atypical antipsychotic drug along with any diabetes medication, you'll be told to monitor closely because "atypical antipsychotics may cause hyperglycemia." You'll get the same warning whether you query for Zyprexa (olanzapine) or Geodon—antipsychotics with very different metabolic profiles.

There are several proprietary drug interaction databases for purchase, such as Lexicomp, Mobile Micromedex, and iFacts. In addition, many EHRs (electronic health records) include drug interactions software. Some studies have compared the various products, and the consensus seems to be that you get what you pay for. For example, in one study the authors ran 40 clinically important and 40 clinically unimportant drug interaction pairs through nine different commercially available programs. They evaluated the results based on both accuracy and ease of use.

The top two overall performers were iFacts and Lexi-Interact. The two free packages that they evaluated performed poorly in this ranking: Mobile PDR was last and Epocrates came in seventh. (Barrons R, *Am J Health Syst Pharm* 2004;61(4):380–385). Of course, this study is old, so you may want to check out the various options for yourself before deciding that it's worth paying for something that you can get for free.

In order to make learning about drug interactions fun, I suggest you purchase the book, *Drug-Drug Interaction Primer: A Compendium of Case Vignettes for the Practicing Clinician* (APPI, 2007), by Neil Sandson. Dr. Sandson's fascinating case vignettes bring an otherwise abstract topic to life.

The Carlat System for Keeping Track of Drug Interactions

When your only task is to look up an interaction between two or more specific drugs, computer software is perfectly adequate.

But more often than not, this is not the kind of data I need while I'm making medication decisions. Most of the time during psychopharm visits, I'm sifting through a mental list of many different candidate medications that I might potentially use for a patient.

For example, in the case of patients with comorbid anxiety and depression, I will typically be entertaining a list of 10 or 20 different medications that might be helpful. Assuming that the patient is already taking two or three meds (psychiatric and non-psychiatric), there will be dozens of possible interactions. As different drug options pop into my mind, I don't particularly want to have to type in the various possible combinations, only to find an excessively long list of "potential" interactions that may not actually be clinically significant. Instead, I would prefer to have a couple of very well organized charts that lay all the information out graphically.

Most of the drug interaction charts I've seen are categorized by P450 enzyme family rather than by medication. I don't organize my clinical thinking in terms of 2D6s and 3A4s; instead, I organize my thinking in terms of drug classes and specific members of those classes. Thus, the most useful chart for me is an alphabetical list of commonly used psychiatric medications, with information about how "clean" or "dirty" each one is in combination with other drugs.

I've created this type of chart, **"Psychiatric Drug Interactions by Medication,"** listed in the Appendix. I've listed all the meds that psychiatrists commonly prescribe in alphabetical order, organized by drug class. I also created a more abbreviated chart for common non-psychiatric medications, also in the Appendix.

Here's an example of how you can use this chart. Let's assume you have a patient on Depakote for bipolar disorder. One day he comes into your office with racing thoughts and mild paranoia. Aside from reviewing his Depakote level and considering a dosage increase, you decide to prescribe one of the atypical antipsychotics, most of which are FDA-approved for treating manic episodes. But you want to avoid prescribing anything that will affect your patient's Depakote level. You could pull out your iPhone and input Depakote along with each of the several antipsychotics you might prescribe—or, you could quickly glance at the Interactions Chart under Depakote and look at the "Watch out for" column. There you'll see that the only clinically relevant interaction is that Depakote increases levels of Lamictal—not an issue in this case, since your patient is not taking Lamictal. Just to be sure, you can then look at the antipsychotic section of the chart, and you'll see that the atypicals do not inhibit or induce the metabolism of any other psychiatric drugs. So you're in the clear, and you can go ahead and prescribe your atypical of choice knowing that it will not mess with your patient's Depakote levels.

But this chart is not enough—there are times when it is, in fact, helpful to have a chart organized by enzymes. This is particularly important when you need to know not only whether the drug you are prescribing will affect the levels of other drugs, but whether its own level will be altered by drugs that your patient is already taking. This is why the column in the Psychiatric Drug Interactions chart labeled "substrate of..." is important. This tells you what enzyme system(s) are primarily responsible for metabolizing that medication. You then need to look up that enzyme system, to see what drugs affect it. For this you want a drug interactions chart organized by enzyme systems. My own version of this standard drug interactions chart, **"Psychiatric Drug Interactions by Enzyme Family"** is printed in the Appendix.

Suppose that you have a patient with schizophrenia who has been maintained on Seroquel, but now is suffering major depression. He is already somewhat sedated on the Seroquel, so you want to make sure that whatever you prescribe will not increase Seroquel levels. Seroquel is metabolized primarily by 3A4 (at least that's what the chart says), so you look at the list of antidepressants to see if any of them affect 3A4. The only ones that do are fluvoxamine and Serzone. You forego those, and prescribe Zoloft.

How to Use the Non-Psychiatric Medication Chart

This is pretty self-explanatory—it's just a list of the more common non-psychiatry meds your patients might be taking, along with corresponding interactions to watch out for.

For example, you are prescribing an elderly woman Celexa and Ativan for panic disorder. She comes in to a visit and announces that her primary care doctor just started her on Zestril (lisinopril) for hypertension. She wants to know if it's OK to take this with your meds. You refer to the "Non-Psych" chart, look up Zestril under "Cardiac Meds," and learn that Zestril' s only significant psychiatric interaction is an increase in lithium levels. You assure your patient that she can go ahead and fill the new prescription.

A Few Tips on How to Use the "Carlat Charts" in Your Office

1. Just because an interaction is listed doesn't mean that it will necessarily cause clinical problems for your patient. According to Neil Sandson, only 10% to 20% of patients will be unlucky enough to develop clinical consequences when

prescribed interacting drugs. But those are still high enough odds to be vigilant.

2. Focus on interactions involving drugs with serious potential toxicity. Among psychiatric drugs, these include cardiac risks with tricyclics, Geodon, and Orap (pimozide); seizure risk with Wellbutrin and Clozaril; risk of confusion and lethargy with lithium; and risk of serious rash with Lamictal. Varying levels of other drugs can cause unpleasant side effects or impaired efficacy, but not catastrophic medical events.

3. When starting a patient on a potent enzyme inhibitor, consider cutting the dose of a vulnerable drug in half right away, since inhibitory effects occur immediately.

4. When starting a patient on a potent enzyme inducer (such as Tegretol), find out if she is on a drug vulnerable to induction (in the case of Tegretol, a 3A4 substrate). If so, wait one to two weeks before increasing the dosage of that drug, because it takes inducers about that long to rev up the production of extra P450 enzymes.

5. When a medication is listed as being the substrate of multiple enzymes, chances are that no inhibiting drug will increase its level much, since if one enzyme is impaired, there are others to take over. (An exception to this rule are the tricyclics, whose metabolism is significantly inhibited by some SSRIs that inhibit several enzymes.) This moderating effect of multiple enzymes doesn't apply when the other drug is an inducer, however, because a single supercharged enzyme can chew up substrate quickly, even while other enzymes systems are sitting around and yawning.

A Short List of What You Really Need to Know

The following alphabetically listed drugs (in one case, a fruit juice) significantly *increase* the levels of a number of other psychiatric and non-psychiatric drugs:

- Depakote
- Grapefruit juice
- Fluvoxamine
- Paxil
- Prozac
- Serzone
- Zoloft (in high doses)

The following drugs significantly *decrease* the levels of other drugs:

- **Tegretol**
- **Smoked tobacco (does not affect nicotine replacement therapy)**
- **St. John's wort**

Protein Binding: Can We Finally Forget About It?

There's been a long-standing debate about the clinical relevance of "protein binding." Many drugs latch onto proteins in the bloodstream, and it is only the unbound fraction of the drug that can actually have a biological effect. A newly prescribed drug with a higher affinity for a particular protein can displace an existing drug, which means that the effective level of the existing drug could increase and cause toxicity.

While all this makes sense, it turns out that there are very few situations in which protein binding has a clinically significant effect on serum levels of medications—at least for medications that psychiatrists are likely to prescribe. According to a 2013 review article, usefully entitled "The Clinical Relevance of Plasma Protein Binding Changes," the only situation in which these effects are significant are when you are working in an intensive care unit and dosing certain types of antibiotics (Roberts JA et al, *Clin Pharmacokinet* 2013;52(1):1–8). Apparently, most changes in unbound fractions caused by competing drugs are relatively minor, and any excess unbound drug tends to go right into its metabolic pathway and is eliminated before it can cause toxicity.

However, changes in free fractions of drugs can cause confusion when you order serum drug levels. Generally, when you order a serum drug level, the lab reports the level of both the bound and the unbound medication. In patients with decreased albumin, or who are taking a competing protein-bound drug, the free fraction will be increased, at least until the extra amount of unbound drug can be processed. If you were to order a drug serum level, however, it would not appear to be high, since the higher free fraction is balanced by the lower bound fraction. In such cases, you can specifically order a "free fraction" of a drug, which will give you a more accurate reading.

Even though there are controversies regarding the importance of protein binding interactions, it's still worth reviewing how protein binding is *theoretically* relevant in psychiatry.

There are four drugs that we psychiatrists commonly prescribe that are highly protein bound:

- Prozac

- Paxil

- Zoloft

- Depakote

While these drugs can displace a variety of other protein-bound drugs, we only need to be concerned about those with a narrow therapeutic index (because in these cases it really matters if there is suddenly too much free drug in the body).

There are three commonly prescribed examples of protein-bound drugs with narrow therapeutic indices:

- Coumadin

- Digox (digoxin)

- Dilantin (phenytoin)

If you have patients taking any of these drugs, the easiest solution is to prescribe something that is not highly protein bound—among SSRIs: Celexa and Lexapro. But if a patient has only responded well to one of the protein-bound psychiatric drugs, you need to watch for signs of toxicity in the other drugs, and it would be prudent to inform the patient's other prescriber that you are adding a drug that may cause an interaction.

These are some common signs of toxicity you should watch for:

Coumadin:
- elevated PT (prothrombin time)
- new onset bruising or bleeding
- hematuria (phenytoin)
- nose bleeds
- dark stools
- acute headache (potential sign of hemorrhagic stroke)

Digox:
- nausea and vomiting
- poor energy
- heart failure
- cardiac arrhythmia

Dilantin:
- hypertrophy of the gums
- ataxia
- nystagmus (involuntary eye movement)

Section II

Special Topics

Chapter 7

Prescribing for
the Elderly and the Young

As if life weren't complicated enough for a hard-working psychopharmacologist these days, we have to add yet another factor to our decision-making—the fact that various aspects of the drug-metabolism process vary with age.

We'll start at the end of the story, that is, with the elderly, because we know so much more about drug metabolism in this age group. The elderly receive much more medical treatment than the young, which has led to a larger body of research published on drug disposition in elderly patients. Psychopharmacologic treatment of children is in its infancy, and we will surely have more to say about psychiatric drug metabolism in this group in years to come.

Drug Metabolism in the Elderly

Absorption. Drug absorption does not get impeded in a predictable way in the elderly, even though there are age-related decreases in GI function, including decreased numbers of intestinal absorptive cells. Because there are so many extra villi to go around, some loss in villi doesn't usually result in a significant effect. Nonetheless, about one out of 20 elderly persons are estimated to have significant problems with drug absorption. These particular patients may come to your attention if they do not seem to be responding to adequate doses of medication. You can always obtain a serum level simply to see if a decent amount is getting into the bloodstream, even if the serum level is not correlated with clinical effect. (For more details on changes in metabolism due to aging, see "Pharmacotherapy in the Elderly," chapter in *Principles and Practice of Geriatric Psychiatry* by Agronin and Maletta, Eds. 2nd ed. Philadelphia, PA: Lippincott Williams & Wilkins; 2011.)

Many drug companies now offer orally dissolving tablets (ODTs), such as FazaClo (rapidly dissolving clozapine), Aricept ODT (donepezil), Klonopin wafers, Risperdal M-Tabs (risperidone), and Zyprexa Zydis (see full list of available ODTs in table below). These formulations dissolve in a matter seconds on the tongue and because they don't need to be taken with water, they are typically marketed as having the advantages of convenience and discretion (for those times when you need to secretly pop a pill during an important meeting, for example).

Theoretically, these formulations would be absorbed more

Psychiatric Medications Available in ODT (Orally Disintegrating Tablet) Form

Medication	ODT Version (Brand Name Unless Specified "G" for Generic)
Alprazolam	Niravam
Aripiprazole	Abilify Discmelt
Clonazepam	Clonazepam ODT (G), Klonopin Wafers
Donepezil	Aricept ODT
Zolpidem	Edluar
Clozapine	FazaClo
Lamotrigine	Lamictal ODT
Mirtazapine	Mirtazapine ODT (G), Remeron SolTab
Risperidone	Risperdal M-Tab
Asenapine	Saphris (both are ODTs)
Olanzapine	Zyprexa Zydis

quickly and dependably because some portion of the pill would be absorbed in the mouth before reaching the GI tract. This, in turn, allows some of the dose to avoid the first pass effect in the liver (which we discussed earlier in Chapter 2). Whether this effect is significant depends on the drug and on how quickly your patients swallow the disintegrating disc.

Dissolving pills are helpful for a variety of patients, including:

- Elderly patients who suffer dysphagia, or difficulty swallowing. Dysphagia is primarily a disease of the elderly, caused by such conditions as stroke, Parkinson's disease, and poorly fitting dentures. So a reasonable question to add to your interview of elderly patients is whether they have swallowing problems; and, if they do, then ask them if they would prefer an orally disintegrating medication.

- Any patient with a swallowing phobia or refusal, including children and involuntarily committed psychiatric patients.

- Patients who have a medical condition causing nausea, since ODTs are less likely to trigger a gagging response.

Distribution. As people age, they tend to lose muscle mass at the expense of adipose tissue (fat). This biological fact can have a significant effect on how we should dose medications in the elderly. To explain why this is so, we have to discuss the dreaded topic of volume of distribution (Vd).

Vd is defined according to the equation:

$$Vd = \frac{\text{Total amount of drug in the body}}{\text{Concentration of drug in the bloodstream}}$$

You can tell by scrutinizing this equation that a very high Vd implies that there is relatively little drug in the bloodstream, which means that there is less drug available to accomplish its therapeutic task. On the other hand, a very low Vd means that there is plenty of medication available.

The concept of Vd has confused medical students through the ages, because a "high Vd" sounds like it should mean that there's a lot of medication in the patient's system. But in fact, a high Vd means that the drug is widely distributed in lots of biological tissues and therefore is *less* plentiful in the blood.

So where does all this drug go if not in the bloodstream?

Primarily in the adipose tissue. Recall from Chapter 5 that most drugs are lipophilic, so they tend to dissolve in fatty tissue. Because the elderly have a higher proportion of fat, lipophilic drugs tend to exit the bloodstream more quickly in these older patients and get stored in adipose tissue, where they are unavailable to act therapeutically in the brain.

Thus with initial doses of drugs, plasma levels may actually be *lower* in the elderly than in younger patients. The catch, however, is that because the drug is stored in fat, it stays around longer, meaning that its effective half-life is longer. Combine this with the fact that the rate of clearance of drugs is often lower in the elderly (due to factors such as decreased blood flow to the liver and decreased glomerular filtration rate), and you can have a real problem with excess accumulation of drugs in elderly patients. (For more details on drug metabolism in the elderly, see the excellent, though somewhat dated, chapter, "Psychotropic Drug Metabolism in Old Age: Principles and Problems of Assessment," in *Psychopharmacology: The Fourth Generation of Progress* by von Moltke LL et al, published online at http://bit.ly/1wUHGpl.)

The preceding few paragraphs help to explain a common clinical phenomenon in treating elderly patients with benzodiazepines. When starting benzos for anxiety or insomnia in the elderly, you might find that these patients don't respond to the very tiny doses with which we are taught to start. This is because the first few doses are whisked away into the patients' fat, rendering the medication less available and causing it to have a briefer duration of effect. However, with repeated dosing, the fat stores get saturated, and benzo levels build up, such that a couple of weeks after starting treatment, these patients may develop signs of benzo toxicity, such as sedation, cognitive impairment, and balance problems.

Thus, particularly in the overweight elderly, rather than "start low, go slow," a more rational approach would be to "start normal, then reduce the dose." This same argument can be applied to obese individuals of any age, although there tends to be less accumulation in younger patients because their liver and kidney functions are more robust.

Biotransformation. All things deteriorate with age, livers and kidneys as much as car engines and roof shingles. Recall that most of the body's biotransformation of drugs occurs in the liver. As we age, the blood flow to the liver decreases, so that at age 65, 45% less blood courses through the liver than at age 25. While this certainly causes some cell death, the liver was cleverly engineered with a redundancy of hepatocytes to ensure that it can continue to function pretty well into old age.

However, the decreased blood flow to the liver does affect first pass metabolism. Recall that in the first pass effect, drug molecules are transported from the intestine directly to the liver (they do not pass either "go" or the brain first), and the liver immediately extracts and deactivates a certain percentage of those molecules. If only half as much blood gets to the liver, a lower proportion of drug molecules will be extracted, leading to a higher spike in drug serum levels. Some drugs, such as benzodiazepines, show only a limited first pass effect: only 10% to 20% of the total is extracted by the liver on first pass, meaning that at least 80% enters general circulation. Thus, for benzodiazepines, a decrement in the first pass extraction does not increase serum concentrations significantly (nonetheless, decreased liver metabolism will prolong these drugs' half-lives). Many other drugs, however, including most antidepressants and antipsychotics, are about 50% extracted on first pass, so less liver blood flow can cause a much higher peak serum concentration than normal.

In addition to decreased hepatic blood flow, some of the P450 (Phase I) enzymes become sluggish in the elderly. Most notably for psychiatry, the 3A4 system slows down. Happily, the 2D6 system, responsible for metabolizing many psychotropics, tends to be unaffected by age. (See the chart in the Appendix for psychiatric drugs metabolized primarily by 2D6.)

Interestingly, Phase II metabolism, in which molecules such as glucuronic acid are attached to drugs to make them water soluble, is not affected by aging at all. In practical terms, this means that drugs that are metabolized mainly by glucuronidation, such as Ativan, Restoril, and Serax (oxazepam), are cleared efficiently in the elderly. Because of the Vd factors cited previously, you still should dose these drugs cautiously, but at least you don't have to worry about a slow liver further lengthening the half-life of these agents.

Excretion and the Aging Kidneys. On average, renal mass declines by 45% by age 80, and there are corresponding declines in renal function. But despite this glum statistic, about a third of the healthy elderly maintain essentially normal kidney function.

Decrements in kidney function are relevant mostly for those very few psychiatric drugs that are metabolized primarily by the kidneys—lithium, Lyrica (pregabalin), and Neurontin. None of these drugs are affected by the liver; but if kidney excretion is impaired, the serum levels will be higher and the drugs' half-lives longer.

Many other drugs are *metabolized* by the liver and then largely *excreted* by the kidneys, but as long as the liver metabolism has rendered the drugs inactive, impaired kidney function will not significantly increase serum levels of the active drug. The exception is those medications that have active metabolites, such as Prozac.

How does one tell if a patient has impaired renal function? If a patient has significant renal disease, this will show up as elevations in the standard renal blood test—the creatinine level. But what about the healthy elderly patient without frank renal disease? Chances are that his or her kidney clearance is lower than it used to be, based on normal age-related declines alone.

Unfortunately, you can't tell how well an elderly person's kidneys are working just by ordering a creatinine level because creatinine is a by-product of muscle tissue and, as we have seen already, muscle mass decreases in the elderly. Thus the kidneys' decreased clearance of creatinine is offset by the decreased production of creatinine in the elderly. For this reason, a normal blood creatinine level may not be informative.

There is a way of measuring the kidneys' specific ability to clear creatinine, called the creatinine clearance test, but this involves collecting a patient's urine for 24 hours, a cumbersome process that most patients refuse unless absolutely necessary. However, there is a way to approximate creatinine clearance from serum creatinine by using the following formula, which takes into account the patient's age, weight, and blood creatinine level(this is the equation for men; for women, multiply result by 0.85):

$$\text{Creatinine Clearance} = \frac{(140 - \text{age in years}) \times (\text{body weight in kg})}{72 \times \text{serum creatinine level}}$$

You might be wondering if all this is more information than you really need to know as a psychiatrist. It may well be. The only time you would try to estimate the creatinine clearance is when you can't figure out why a patient's serum lithium level is very high in the presence of a very low dose. But chances are you would refer such a patient to his or her primary care physician for a complete work-up.

Protein Binding. What about protein binding and the elderly? In the absence of malnutrition or chronic GI problems, serum protein levels are not typically decreased in the elderly. And as we discussed in Chapter 6, drug interactions involving protein binding are generally not significant because any excess free fraction of a medication gets metabolized via normal routes. However, if your elderly patient has impaired hepatic metabolism, protein binding interactions could result in sustained high serum levels of certain drugs.

The Bottom Line: How Should You Dose Drugs in the Elderly? The effects of aging on drug metabolism are complicated. Some factors, such as decreased hepatic first pass extraction, decreased P450 activity, and decreased renal clearance, act to *increase* **serum** levels of medications. Other factors, such as a higher Vd, tend to *decrease* serum levels, while at the same time increasing the half-lives of the drugs. Add to this the unpredictable intra-individual variation in patients' biology, and you have a very confusing situation on your hands!

Thus, ultimately, the tried-and-true dictum applies in prescribing for the elderly: "Start low, go slow." While this won't be true for all patients or for all drugs you have little to lose by hewing to this practice, whereas you can easily cause catastrophic outcomes with too aggressive dosing.

What does "start low, go slow" mean in actual practice? A good rule of thumb is to start at half the standard adult dose and to titrate upwards at half your standard rate.

Drug Metabolism in the Young

My focus in this section is on the toddler age group and above, because few psychiatrists are prescribing drugs for infants. This simplifies the job considerably, because most of the really complicated differences in drug metabolism occur only in the very, very young.

The bottom line in prescribing for children is that you have to decrease doses of most psychiatric drugs in proportion to the lower weight of a given pediatric patient. This may not be a big news flash to most prescribers; nor is it necessarily obvious, because some of us may well wonder whether a child's young and supple metabolic machinery might chew up drugs faster, so as to compensate for his or her lower weight. In general, this isn't true, though there are some exceptions, so read on.

Absorption. A child's GI tract absorbs drugs similarly to that of an adult. Some authorities (see reference in next section) mention that the transit time of drugs in the GI tract of children tends to be shorter, which may have a particular effect on the absorption of extended-release medication. For example, research has shown that Theochron (extended-release theophylline) is more unpredictably absorbed in children than in adults.

The implication is that extended-release versions of psychostimulants, such as Adderall XR and Concerta, may be pushed through a child's GI tract too quickly to allow absorption of every last anti-ADHD molecule, resulting in a duration of effect shorter than you might predict. You can compensate for such problems either by increasing the dose of the extended-release version or by switching to an immediate-release form of the medication.

Biotransformation and Excretion. Children and adults share the same collection of Phase I and Phase II enzymes, but liver metabolism works a bit faster in children, at least until adolescence. Similarly, kidney filtration is faster in children. Both of these factors mean that, at least for some kids and for some drugs, dosing ends up being higher than what might be expected based on weight alone.

The main example of this is in prescribing lithium to children. Most studies of lithium for bipolar disorder or aggressive behavior in children (ages six to 12) have reported that doses up to 1500 mg/day were required to reach adequate serum lithium levels. The same more aggressive dosing might be needed for both Neurontin and Lyrica, because both of these are excreted unchanged by the kidneys.

By adolescence, drug metabolism slows way down and approaches normal adult levels. Thus if you follow a patient from childhood into adolescence, you may actually need to decrease the dose of medication as the child becomes a teenager. (For more detailed information on the peculiarities of drug metabolism in children, see both: Benedetti MS & Baltes EL *Fundam Clin Pharmacol* 2003;17(3):281–299; and more recently, de Wildt SN et al, *Arch Dis Child* 2014;99:1137–1142.)

Chapter 8

Pharmacodynamic Drug Interactions

Pharmacodynamic interactions in psychiatry refer to ways in which one drug affects another drug's action on neurotransmitter (NT) systems. In this chapter, we'll focus on three of the most potentially dangerous pharmacodynamic interactions in psychiatry: those related to monoamine oxidase inhibitors (MAOI), serotonin syndrome (SS), and anticholinergics.

The MAOI-Cheese Interaction: Some Historical Perspective

Perhaps the most dreaded side effect in all of psychiatry is the MAOI-cheese interaction. But for several years after MAOIs were introduced, nobody had an inkling of this potential danger. In 1961, a case report was published in the *Lancet* of a woman who died of a subarachnoid hemorrhage while taking Parnate (tranylcypromine), but because these events occurred often enough in patients not taking MAOIs, clinicians were slow to blame Parnate.

It took a psychiatric resident to save the day. Barry Blackwell, who was training at Maudsley Hospital in London at the time, began reading about sporadic cases of high blood pressure, headache, and subarachnoid hemorrhages in patients taking MAOIs. A pharmacist told Blackwell that the pharmacist's wife, who was taking an MAOI, had developed two episodes of hypertension and headache after eating cheese. Intrigued, Blackwell and a colleague experimented on themselves: they took Parnate for a week, then gorged on cheese. They felt perfectly fine. Nonetheless, Blackwell consulted on several cases in his hospital of patients taking MAOIs who developed hypertensive headaches after eating cheese sandwiches. He published his suspicions in the *Lancet* in 1963, but it still took some time before a skeptical medical community took this MAOI-cheese connection seriously, partly because there was no known mechanism to explain it. (For more details and references related to this story, see the fascinating book *The Anti-Depressant Era* by David Healy, Harvard University Press, 1997.)

This historical aside is interesting because it affords some perspective on the dangers of MAOI interactions. MAOIs were prescribed frequently for several years by physicians who had no knowledge of possible drug or food interactions, and yet the rate of fatal reactions was extremely low. With our current knowledge of these interactions, the risk of serious problems is even lower.

The MAOI-Tyramine Interaction: The Mechanism Explained

MAOIs, as their name implies, cause the enzyme monoamine oxidase (MAO) to be inactivated. MAO comes in two forms: the A form and the B form. MAO-A is the troublesome molecule in this story, because its normal function is to metabolize and break down the neurotransmitters (NTs) serotonin, norepinephrine (NE), and to some extent dopamine (DA). Thus, Parnate, Nardil (phenelzine), and Marplan (isocarboxazid) increase levels of all three of these NTs by inhibiting MAO-A.

These changes in NT levels ease both depressive and anxiety symptoms, and MAOI side effects are generally fairly tolerable—insomnia or sedation, orthostatic dizziness, lowered libido, and occasional weight gain. When no dangerous interactions enter the equation, MAOIs are tolerated better than tricyclic antidepressants (TCAs) and a bit worse than SSRIs, and are considered by some authorities to be more effective than either type for depression with atypical features (see, for example, APA's *Practice Guidelines for the Treatment of Patients with Major Depressive Disorder, Third Edition,* available at http://bit.ly/1vfiPwe).

Enter cheese. Certain cheeses, in addition to several other foods and beverages, contain high quantities of the amino acid tyramine. Why is tyramine so potentially troublesome?

To answer that, it's helpful to know that tyramine is produced from another amino acid, tyrosine. Tyrosine is (or should be) quite famous among psychiatrists, because it is the precursor of both DA and NE. The synthetic pathway that you learned in basic biochemistry is:

$$Tyrosine \rightarrow DOPA \rightarrow Dopamine \rightarrow Norepinephrine$$

The action of NE is terminated by MAO-A, as well as by another enzyme, catechol-O-methyl transferase. By a separate pathway, tyrosine can also be transformed to tyramine, which, like NE, is broken down by MAO-A. At this point, you might be thinking that because MAOIs prevent tyramine's breakdown, this leads to a buildup of tyramine's precursor, tyrosine, leading to too much DA and NE via the synthetic pathway outlined above.

While this roundabout mechanism is part of the story, the major way that excess tyramine causes high blood pressure is via a more immediate effect on NE. Tyramine is sometimes termed a "false neurotransmitter" because it gets actively transported into neurons and displaces NE, increasing NE levels in the blood stream (Meck JV et al, *J Cardiovasc Pharmacol* 2003;41(1):126–131). This, in turn, can result in vasoconstriction and hypertension. In fact, when volunteers (not taking MAOIs) ingest large amounts of tyramine, they experience a small rise in blood pressure, because it takes a little while for the body's MAO to metabolize this extra tyramine (VanDenBerg CM et al, *J Clin Pharmacol* 2003;43(6):604–609).

Now imagine dumping tyramine into a body that does not have any functioning MAO. This is the situation of a patient on MAOIs. In this case, there is a double whammy of NE. First, the MAOI inhibits the breakdown of NE directly; and second, the tyramine, acting as an independent false neurotransmitter, displaces NE from nerve terminals (see the figure on the next page). The combined effect floods the body with NE, causing vasoconstriction, severe hypertension, and potentially catastrophic sequelae such as stroke.

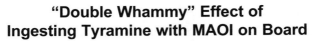

"Double Whammy" Effect of Ingesting Tyramine with MAOI on Board

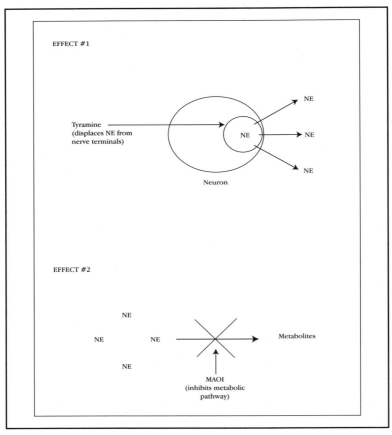

How do foods get to be high in tyramine? Via the action of bacteria on tyrosine, which is found in high amounts in many high protein foods. Bacteria such as *Enterococcus* and *Lactobacillus* contain tyrosine decarboxylase, which converts tyrosine to tyramine. Hence, foods that: (1) contain amino acids (eg, have protein); and (2) have a lot of bacteria in them are precisely those foods that are likely to be loaded with tyramine. One of the best ways for bacteria to grow is by allowing food to sit around for a long time, which is why aged foods of all sorts are on the high-tyramine list—stinky cheeses, smoked meats, overly ripe foods such as bananas and avocados, and fermented liquids (beer, certain wines, soy sauce). This is also why we tell patients on MAOIs to eat foods when they are fresh. The longer cheese or meat is left in the fridge, the more bacteria, and hence the more tyramine.

Because tyramine content varies so drastically depending on freshness, some foods that have in the past been considered absolutely contraindicated are now widely considered safe if consumed when they are fresh. A group of researchers at the University of Toronto has taken the lead in actually measuring the tyramine content of foods commonly contraindicated and published the findings in several papers. They found, for example, that major food-chain pizzas had safe quantities of tyramine, including a Domino's double-cheese, double-pepperoni pizza (Shulman KI & Walker SE, *J Clin Psychiatry* 1999;60(3):191–193). The serving sizes were liberal: a half of a medium pizza. Because most pizzas are made with fresh mozzarella, which, while aged, contains little tyramine, it appears that patients taking MAOIs can indeed enjoy pizza dinners, at least when they are made fresh to order and when the only cheese they contain is mozzarella. Note that some gourmet pizzas may contain other, more flavorful (and thus more aged and higher in tyramine) cheeses and should be avoided (Feinberg S & Holzer B, [letter] *J Clin Psychiatry* 2000;61(2):145). (For a comprehensive recent update on dietary restrictions and MAOIs, see Flockhart DA, *J Clin Psychiatry* 2012;73(suppl1):17–24.)

The MAOI Diet

Foods to absolutely avoid:
  • Aged cheeses: cheddar, fontina, brie, blue, camembert, muenster, swiss (note: patients might get lucky and eat specific servings of these cheeses that have very little tyramine, but the content is so unpredictable that they should all be avoided)

- Tap beer

- Fava beans

- Sauerkraut

- Some aged, cured, or smoked meats, such as air-dried sausage, pastrami, salami, bologna, pepperoni in large amounts (although it seems safe in chain restaurant pizzas, see below)

Foods that are quite risky but if patients really can't live without them, and don't mind playing a little Russian roulette with their blood pressure, can be eaten with caution:

- Tofu (must be extremely fresh; that is, made either the day it is consumed or the day before and stored well)

- Soy sauce (no more than about three teaspoons or so per day, meaning that the only safe way to have soy sauce is to add it yourself, as Chinese restaurants may well add much more than this in a serving)

- Miso soup

Foods that are a little risky, but probably safe in general:

- Cheese pizzas made with mozzarella (even pizzas with pepperoni and mozzarella are probably safe if they come from a reputable restaurant chain that serves fresh food)

Foods that are safe:

- These cheeses: mozzarella, American, cottage, ricotta, cream

- Other dairy products: yogurt, milk, cream

- Alcohol: wine, bottled beers, most hard liquors (some authorities recommend avoiding red wine, but it appears that red wine contains very low levels of tyramine and that the famous "red wine headache" that many people (on or off MAOIs) report has nothing to do with the tyramine content of red wine—see article in Littlewood JT et al, *Lancet* 1988;331(8585):558–559)

- Chocolate (some authorities recommend "caution" in eating chocolate because it contains caffeine and can theoretically cause hypertension in combinations with MAOIs, but this is apparently a problem only in very high quantities)

MAOIs and Serotonin Syndrome

While the tyramine interaction leading to hypertension is the most famous and feared MAOI interaction, serotonin syndrome (SS) is probably more common. In fact, the most infamous case involving MAOIs, the Libby Zion case in New York, involved a death due to SS, in which an MAOI was combined with Demerol (meperidine), causing malignant hyperthermia and death due to cardiac arrest.

An interesting aside to the Libby Zion case is that it resulted in the formation of a New York State government commission, the Bell Commission, to investigate the work hours of medical residents. This was because the medical intern who had been called about Zion's agitation had been awake for 18 hours when paged. Rather than thoroughly investigating the cause of the agitation, the intern ordered restraints and a dose of Haldol (haloperidol). Presumably, a less sleep-deprived intern might have instituted measures to prevent Zion's death. Eventually, the commission's findings led to a law limiting resident's work hours to 80 hours per week (for more background, see http://nyti.ms/11qiXQJ).

SS is best thought of as serotonin *toxicity*, and it occurs on a spectrum, from barely recognizable to potentially lethal. Because it is the result of the body becoming overwhelmed by serotonin, one of the major causes of SS is serotonin reuptake inhibitor (SRI) overdose. But SRI overdose alone rarely, if ever, causes death. Deaths due to SS are generally caused by *combination* overdoses, one of the most common being the MAOI-SRI combination.

Recall that MAO-A normally breaks down both NE and serotonin. Stimulating the serotonin system in this way is therapeutic. But if another source of serotonin is added, the body is unable to process it due to MAO inhibition, and some degree of serotonin toxicity is the result.

The largest database on SS comes from a group of toxicologists that analyzed 2,222 cases of overdose on serotonergic drugs occurring in the Newcastle region of Australia from 1987 to 2002 (Dunkley EJC et al, *QJM* 2003;96(9):635–642). The researchers found that 15% of SSRI overdoses led to SS, whereas fully 50% of combined overdoses of MAOIs and SSRIs led to SS; and in the latter cases, the syndrome was much more severe.

Clinical Symptoms of Serotonin Toxicity and Serotonin Syndrome

There is a wide range in presentation of serotonin syndrome from mild to potentially life threatening. Anyone who prescribes SSRIs regularly sees symptoms of mild to moderate serotonin toxicity, including jitteriness, insomnia, GI disturbances, and cognitive impairment such as word finding difficulties or general "spaciness." We treat such problems by decreasing the SSRI dose and treating the side effects with adjuncts like benzodiazepines or Wellbutrin.

As serotonin toxicity becomes more extreme, it eventually crosses a line and becomes "serotonin syndrome." The classic diagnostic triad includes *autonomic symptoms,* such as hyperthermia, hypertension, and shivering; *neuromuscular symptoms,* such as tremor, hyperreflexia, and restlessness; and *cognitive symptoms,* such as confusion and agitation. Of all of these symptoms, the most reliable for accurately diagnosing SS are the neuromuscular symptoms, such as clonus (rapid alternating relaxation and contractions of muscles, often measured by flexing the patient's foot and watching for rhythmic contractions of the ankle), hyperreflexia, and muscular rigidity (for a good review, see Volpi-Abadie J et al, *Ochsner J* 2013;13(4): 533–540).

Unlike neuroleptic malignant syndrome (NMS), which also presents with autonomic instability, mental status changes, and rigidity, SS is rapidly progressive and includes hyperreflexia as well as rigidity. (For a brief synopsis of the differences between SS and NMS, see Gillman KP, [letter] *J Clin Psychopharm* 2005;25(6):625–626).

A Controversial Issue: How Relevant Is Serotonin Syndrome in Clinical Practice?

While there is no disagreement in the field about the fact that SS exists and can be deadly, there is much controversy about how common it is and which drug combinations cause it. As in any controversial point in medicine, there are different "factions" arguing their points—an inclusive faction (arguing that SS is more common and less predictable than appreciated) and a purist faction (arguing that SS occurs primarily in clear situations of serotonin toxicity).

The inclusive faction published a review article on SS in the *New England Journal of Medicine* (Boyer EW & Shannon M, *N Engl J Med* 2005;352(11):1112–1120) and included a table listing dozens of drugs "associated with the serotonin syndrome." Included in the list were almost all antidepressant medications. Even more intimidating to office-based psychiatrists was the article's warning that "a single therapeutic dose of an SSRI has caused the serotonin syndrome."

If you track down the reference for this statement (Gill M et al, *Ann Emerg Med* 1999;33(4):457–459), you will find that the case report in question was of an 11-year-old boy whose diagnosis was reported as "ADHD" but who was inexplicably being treated with Trilafon (perphenazine) and Cogentin (benztropine), along with Depakote (which had been recently discontinued). He was then prescribed Luvox; and one hour after ingesting his first dose of 50 mg (double the usual starting dose of 25 mg in children), the patient became agitated and unresponsive. Paramedics brought him to the ER, and over the next 48 hours he was treated in the ICU for hyperthermia, agitation, tremor, and rigidity. Fortunately, the child recovered completely.

This case may very well have been an example of SS, although NMS is a possible alternative because the boy was also taking a neuroleptic. But simply referring to this complex case of pediatric polypharmacy as an example of "a single therapeutic dose of an SSRI" causing SS tells only a small part of the story and is some-what misleading.

There are dozens of case reports in the literature, many impli-cating apparently innocuous dosages of standard antidepressants in life-threatening SS. As valuable as individual cases can be, they are vulnerable to misinterpretation and inappropriate generaliza-tion. In fact, the experts on serotonin toxicity referred to earlier in this chapter (the group that published the analysis of 2,222 cases of overdoses on serotonergic drugs) have made a side career of scouring the literature for misleading case reports of SS and publishing letters of rebuttal. In one illustrative example, an apparent case of SS induced by a therapeutic dose of Ultram was published, but the actual clinical scenario involved a 79-year-old woman who was also taking 75 mg QD of Elavil (amitriptyline) (Kitson R & Carr B, *Anaesthesia* 2005;60(9):934–935). In the rebuttal letter, the writer pointed out that anticholinergic delirium due to Elavil was more likely the cause of her symptoms than SS (Gillman K, *Anaesthesia* 2006;61(1):76).

In the next section, we'll take a hard-nosed look at which medication combinations are most likely to lead to SS.

Specific Drug Combinations: An Evaluation of the Dangers

MAOIs and SSRIs/serotonin-norepinephrine reuptake inhibitors (SNRIs). This is one of the most dangerous combination of medications in psychiatry and should be absolutely avoided. There is still confusion about appropriate washouts when transitioning from one class to another, so here is some clarification.

When switching from an SSRI/SNRI to an MAOI: Wait at least five half-lives before starting an MAOI. The usual rule of thumb is more conservative than five half-lives, and is generally listed as 14 days on the reasonable theory that there may still be some residual reuptake inhibition after all the actual medication has washed out of the patient's system. For the special case of Prozac, you should wait a full five weeks, because the half-lives of the parent drug and its active metabolites are so long. There is actually one case report of a patient who developed SS on Parnate even after a six-week Prozac washout (Coplan JD & Gorman JM, *Am J Psychiatry* 1993;150(5):837). Thus if you want to be extra cautious, wait five weeks after stopping Prozac, then check a norfluoxetine level (the active metabolite), and only start an MAOI if that level is undetectable.

When switching from any MAOI to an SSRI/SNRI: Wait 14 days before starting an SSRI/SNRI. Because most MAOIs have a half-life of 24 hours (or less), a 14-day washout is conservative but takes into account the fact that currently available MAOIs are *irreversible* inhibitors of MAO, meaning that the enzyme is essentially destroyed. After washout, the body needs another week or so to remanufacture enough MAO in order to safely deal with the SSRI/SNRI.

MAOIs and Tricyclics. While the *PDR* contraindicates this combination, that hasn't prevented adventurous clinicians from using it. In an early trial, 17 patients with treatment-resistant depression were randomized to electroconvulsive therapy vs. a combination of Nardil and Elavil. The combination was safe but ineffective (Davidson J et al, *Arch Gen Psychiatry* 1978;35(5):639–642). More recently, 25 patients with treatment-resistant depression were treated with Marplan and Elavil. Patients tolerated it well, and half of them responded (Berlanga C & Ortega-Soto HA, *J Affective Dis* 1995;34(3):187–192). In general, Anafranil (clomipramine) and Tofranil (imipramine) are considered the most dangerous TCAs to combine with MAOIs, and the most dangerous way to combine MAOIs and TCAs is to add a TCA when a patient is already taking an MAOI. Adding an MAOI when a TCA is already on board is less risky, but still must be done with great caution.

MAOIs and Tegretol. MAOIs are officially contraindicated with Tegretol because of a heightened seizure risk, though the mechanism is unclear. Nonetheless, in one report, a series of 10 patients tolerated MAOI augmentation of Tegretol without any adverse events (Ketter TA et al, *J Clin Psychiatry* 1995;56(10):471–475).

MAOIs and Other Antidepressants. MAOIs are contraindicated with Wellbutrin, Remeron (mirtazapine), and Serzone. However, there are no case reports of adverse events with these combinations, so it appears that the contraindications are listed in package inserts by companies wanting to be extra cautious. It's likely that certain patients could tolerate trials of any of these combinations.

MAOIs and Psychostimulants. The *PDR* contraindicates this combination but it is used frequently by clinicians medicating patients with treatment-resistant depression. A recent review of the literature on combining MAOIs with methylphenidate or amphetamine concluded that it is effective and relatively safe (Feinberg SS, *J Clin Psychiatry* 2004;65(11):1520–1524). The few cases of hypertensive crises attributed to this combination were published in the 1960s, and some involved outdated delivery strategies, such as intravenous methylphenidate. Over the last 30 years, no cases of serious adverse events associated with this combination have been published. To prevent problems in your own practice, add stimulants to MAOIs slowly and at low doses, and only to particularly reliable patients.

MAOIs and Pain Relievers. Because several analgesics have significant serotonergic activity, they are contraindicated in combination with MAOIs.

Darvon (propoxyphene): Contraindicated.

Dextromethorphan (contained in Robitussin DM): Contraindicated.

Meperidine (Demerol): Contraindicated. As discussed above, the combination of an MAOI with Demerol apparently led to the death of Libby Zion in 1984.

Methadone: Contraindicated.

Ultram: While there have been no case reports of MAOI/Ultram problems, the Ultram package insert recommends caution.

Triptans (used for migraines): Three triptans are contraindicated with MAOIs: sumatriptan (Imitrex), rizatriptan (Maxalt), and zolmitriptan (Zomig). They are the only triptans that are almost *entirely dependent* on MAO for their metabolism—meaning that an MAOI will cause levels to increase to potentially dangerous levels (Armstrong SC & Cozza KL, *Psychosomatics* 2002;43(6):502–504). Other triptans, namely almotriptan (Axert), naratriptan (Amerge), eletripan (Relpax) and frovitriptan (Frova), are not depending on MAO for metabolism and therefore can be combined with MAOIs with caution (http://bit.ly/1t2OhlS).

The following narcotics can be safely combined with MAOIs: morphine, codeine, OxyContin, buprenorphine (the active ingredient of Suboxone), ibuprofen, aspirin, and acetaminophen.

MAOIs and Miscellaneous Other Drugs. The following drugs have MAOI activity themselves and so should not be combined with MAOIs: Zyvox (linezolid), an antibiotic; selegiline, used in the treatment of Parkinson's disease and now as an antidepressant called EMSAM; and iproniazid, an antituberculous agent. Other potential interactions are with Sinemet (carbidopa-levodopa) and St. John's wort.

SSRIs and Pain Relievers. SSRIs can be combined safely with all analgesics except, possibly, for Ultram and triptans.

Ultram: A recent review described 10 case reports of SS apparently caused by combining serotonergic antidepressants with Ultram (Park SH et al, *J Pharm Prac* 2014;27(1):71–78). The implicated drugs included Celexa, Prozac, Paxil, Zoloft, and Remeron. More than half of these patients were over 65, and in all cases the symptoms resolved after making medication adjustments such as discontinuing either the antidepressant or Ultram or simply decreasing the dose of the antidepressant. The combination is not contraindicated, but you may get phone calls from pharmacists who want to make sure you know about the possible interaction. You can avoid such delays by jotting on your prescription, "Am aware of possible interaction with Ultram; will monitor closely."

Triptans: Until fairly recently, combining triptans with SSRIs was considered relatively safe, as long as patients were monitored for serotonin toxicity (Gardner DM & Lynd LD, *Ann Pharmacother* 1998;32(1):33–38). According to a study of over 240,000 patients who were prescribed triptans, 20% of them were also prescribed SSRIs. Given the vast numbers of patients taking this drug combination, one would think that SS would be well reported if it were a risk, but case reports are scarce. Large-scale studies of triptan use have reported no instances of SS in patients on the combination (see Tepper S et al, *Headache* 2003;43,(1):44–48).

Nonetheless, in July 2006 the FDA announced a public health advisory warning patients and physicians about the potential dangers of this combination (http://1.usa.gov/1EXHNVx). The FDA based this advisory on a review of 29 cases of SS apparently related to combinations of SRIs and triptans. None resulted in death, although two of the cases were described as "life-threatening." Later, the American Headache Society disputed the warning, saying that many of the cases of SS were probably misdiagnosed, and that SSRIs and triptans are in fact not contraindicated (Evans RW et al, *Headache* 2010;50(6):1089–1099).

In the meantime, the FDA continues to review the evidence and may decide to rescind the warning in the future. It is somewhat reassuring that the main culprit in SS is over-stimulation of 5HT2A receptors specifically, whereas triptans are agonists at the 5HT1 receptor. Also, triptans are usually used as occasional rescue drugs to abort migraines, rather than as prophylaxis, meaning that serum levels don't stay high, further decreasing their risk of causing SS.

For the time being, you should document in your chart that you have discussed the risk of SS in patients to whom you have prescribed the combination.

Transdermal Selegiline: A Safer MAOI?

EMSAM (transdermal selegiline) was approved by the FDA in 2008 for depression. By way of background, the *oral* version of selegiline (Eldepryl) is an MAOI that has been used for years in the treatment of Parkinson's disease. It is different from standard MAOIs because it is selective for the MAO-B subtype of MAO at doses of 10 mg or lower. MAO-B is not involved in NT metabolism, nor is it found in the GI tract, so inhibiting it does not lead to negative tyramine effects.

So why isn't Eldepryl used more in depression? Because in order to be effective for depression, the dose has to be quite high — over 30 mg/day (Bodkin JA & Kwon AE, *Psych Ann* 2001;31(6):385–391). At this dose, its selectivity for MAO-B is lost, and it acts like any other MAOI. Nonetheless, many psychiatrists with experience using MAOIs have found high-dose Eldepryl to be quite effective and relatively well-tolerated. Unfortunately, it's more of a hassle to prescribe than the likes of Parnate or Nardil, both because it comes only in 5 mg strength (an inconvenience for patients taking high doses) and because it is quite expensive.

The transdermal patch takes advantage of the fact that the drug is absorbed directly into the bloodstream and does not go through the gut or the liver initially. This, in turn, yields two metabolic benefits. First, because selegiline's concentration in the GI tract is much lower than with the oral version, there is less inhibition of dietary tyramine's metabolism, and so less concern about dietary restrictions. Second, because there is no first pass effect through the liver, a relatively low amount of selegiline can provide therapeutic concentrations in the brain, minimizing systemic side effects.

What all this means is that EMSAM does not require any dietary restrictions, but this is true only at the starting dose of 6 mg/24 hours. At the higher available doses of 9 mg and 12 mg, all the usual restrictions apply, because these doses are considered to be high enough to cause enough MAOI to enter the gut and to inhibit the metabolism of tyramine. However, if you take a look at the raw data used by the FDA to make these crucial dosing decisions, you come away with the sense that they were extremely cautious, and that in fact the 9 mg dose is likely to be quite safe without dietary restrictions. (You can read the FDA hearing transcript at http://1.usa.gov/11hTvNP.) What this means in clinical practice is that you can be somewhat less insistent that patients follow their MAOI diet when they are on EMSAM 9 mg than if they were on the highest dose, 12 mg.

To increase the confusion, the entire discussion above applies only to MAOI-food interactions and not MAOI-drug interactions. EMSAM is considered dangerous to combine with serotonergic drugs at *all* doses, including the 6 mg dose. This is because these drug interactions have nothing to do with tyramine and generally involve excessive serotonin. However, since EMSAM was released, there have been many cases of patients taking supposedly forbidden medications without suffering serotonin syndrome. (For a comprehensive review of EMSAM's safety record, see Asnis GM & Henderson MA, *Neuropsychiatr Dis Treat* 2014;10:1911–1923.)

So, is EMSAM a "safer" MAOI? Probably so, and as we gain more experience using it, we'll all likely become more comfortable with it, which is a good thing for those patients who have failed all the usual antidepressant suspects.

Anticholinergic Drug Interactions

First, recall that there are two parts of the autonomic nervous system: the parasympathetic system and the sympathetic system. The parasympathetic system manages physiological activities during rest, so it is sometimes called the "rest and digest" system. It relies on the neurotransmitter acetylcholine (ACh). In medical school pharmacology courses, many of us learned how ACh affects the body by using the mnemonic "SLUD": Salivation, Lacrimation, Urination, Defecation. In other words, ACh causes drooling, tearing up of the eyes, and facilitates both urination and defecation. I suggest augmenting this with a "C" standing for "Cognition," since ACh is necessary for good cognitive functioning. (This is why our anti-dementia drugs are cholinesterase inhibitors—they inhibit enzymes that break down ACh, causing ACh levels to rise, theoretically pepping up cognition.) By extension, if ACh facilitates SLUD-C, drugs that are *anti*-cholinergic—for example the tricyclics, Paxil, Cogentin, Artane (trihexyphenydil), Benadryl (diphenhydramine), and several antipsychotics—are "Anti-SLUD-C." This means that they cause dry mouth, dry eyes (and blurry vision), urinary retention, constipation, and confusion.

It's a little more complicated, because there are actually two different ACh receptor types: muscarinic receptors, which mediate the SLUD part of SLUD-C, and nicotinic, which mediate the pro-cognitive, or "C" part of the mnemonic.

The key thing to remember as you treat patients is that combining drugs with anticholinergic properties can cause significant problems, especially in the elderly, who are prone to developing confusion and other side effects when overdosed on these drugs. There is an excellent, free, pocket card listing medications with anticholinergic effects on the web at http://bit.ly/1uG0iwv.

On the next page is an abbreviated list of the most commonly prescribed anticholinergic psychiatric drugs. Memorize these, and be aware of the possible additive effects of combining them.

Drugs with Anticholinergic Effects Commonly Prescribed by Psychiatrists

Hydroxyzine (Vistaril)
Diphenhydramine (Benadryl)
Benztropine (Cogentin)
Trihexyphenidyl (Artane)
Paroxetine (Paxil)
Tricyclic antidepressants
Low potency antipsychotics, including Thorazine (chlorpromazine), thioridazine (Mellaril), clozapine (Clozaril), olanzapine (Zyprexa), and quetiapine (Seroquel)

Chapter 9

Generic Medications and Drug Metabolism

Generic drugs are playing an increasingly important role in the practice of psychiatry. Most medications in all categories of therapeutics are now available as generics, including stimulants, antidepressants, atypical antipsychotics, anxiolytics, and mood stabilizers.

The benefits of prescribing generic medications are clear— reduced co-payments for our patients and a reduced overall financial burden on the health care system. But what about the potential disadvantages? Most psychiatrists have either had experience with their own patients or heard stories from colleagues about patients switched from brand to generic formulations who have had break through psychiatric symptoms. The question is, aside from such anecdotal reports, is there scientific evidence documenting the bio-equivalence of generics and brand name medications in psychiatry?

We'll review the research on this topic, but first, it will be helpful to outline the history and current regulations of generics in the United States.

Generic Drugs: A Primer

The story of the modern generic drug industry began in 1984, when Congress passed the Hatch-Waxman Act. This legislation was introduced because of rising pharmaceutical costs, and its purpose was to make it easier for companies to manufacture generic versions of high-priced medications.

When a drug company discovers a new compound, it quickly applies for a series of patents, which last 20 years from the time the compound was first discovered. Of course, a good chunk of a compound's patent life is taken up with all the basic clinical research required to win FDA approval. Companies must first test drugs for safety in animals, then in human volunteers in Phase I trials, then in groups of patients in Phase II trials, and finally in very large groups of patients in Phase III trials. In order to receive FDA approval, companies must provide positive results of at least two large placebo-controlled trials. The drug testing and evaluation process takes an average of 10 years, so that most drugs have only another 10 years of patent protection remaining after FDA approval. Nonetheless, a blockbuster drug can earn billions of dollars in that time span. (See the FDA's Office of Generic Drugs website at http://1.usa.gov/1ujjdM1 for more extensive information.)

Before the Hatch-Waxman Act, generic companies were required to go through the same time consuming Research and Development process as the "originator" companies (the companies that made the original drug discovery). This requirement meant that very few generic medications entered the marketplace, because generic drug companies couldn't possibly recoup their R&D investments by selling low-cost generics.

The Hatch-Waxman legislation changed FDA regulations so that generic companies are now permitted to rely on the originator company's efficacy data. In order to win FDA approval, the generic manufacturer must demonstrate that its copycat product is both chemically and biologically identical to the brand. As a further incentive, the first company to produce a generic version is awarded six months of market exclusivity, meaning that no other generic companies are allowed to compete during that time. This explains why prices of generic drugs take several months to decrease significantly.

Generic Drugs and Bioequivalence

The FDA requires that generic drugmakers demonstrate that the generic is "biologically equivalent" to the brand name drug that it will replace. In order to accomplish this, companies conduct studies in which 25 to 30 healthy volunteers take a single dose of both the brand and generic versions. Their blood is drawn sequentially, and the data are analyzed to obtain averages for Cmax (maximum serum concentration), AUC (area under the curve), half-life, and sometimes other variables. (See Chapter 3 for an explanation of these quantities.) The numbers obtained for the generic are then compared with those obtained for the brand name drug, and this comparison forms the basis for an assessment of the bioequivalence of the two formulations.

FDA guidelines specify that the bioavailability of a generic must be, on average, between 80% and 125% of that of the original brand. Otherwise, the generic will not be approved.

This may seem like a liberal amount of leeway, particularly for drugs that have a narrow therapeutic index, such as anti-seizure medications or anti-arrhythmics. The fact is, however, that most generics achieve much better bioequivalence than this spread suggests. We know this because every few years the FDA reviews all the bioequivalence studies that generic companies have submitted. The last time these data were published, the average difference between the AUC of generic and brand name drugs was reported to be only 3.5% (Davit BM et al, *Ann Pharmacother* 2009;43(10):1583–1597). Thus, the bioavailability of a 50 mg dose of generic sertraline is likely to deviate from 50 mg of Zoloft by no more than about 2 mg either way. A patient who is switched from 50 mg of Zoloft to 50 mg of generic sertraline may actually be absorbing between 48 mg and 52 mg QD—unlikely to be clinically significant in any but the most exquisitely sensitive patients.

The FDA provides a rating of bioequivalence. An "AB" rating means that the generic has been shown to be bioequivalent to the brand name in human studies. An "AA" rating means that no human studies have been done, but the drug is considered inherently unlikely to have bioequivalence problems. Almost all generics are AB rated. About 4% are only B rated, meaning that they may not be bioequivalent. These are generally older drugs that have never been adequately tested. In many states, unless you write "no substitutions" on a prescription, the pharmacist is mandated to fill it as a generic—but only if the generic is AB or AA rated.

Some patients and physicians are concerned that generics might be manufactured overseas in substandard factories. However, the FDA inspects both branded and generic drug factories in order to enforce "good manufacturing practices." In fact, some of the most egregious recent examples of substandard manufacturing practices have occurred in factories producing *branded* medications. For example, in 2005, the FDA ordered GlaxoSmithKline to halt production of Paxil CR at its Puerto Rican facility because defects in the pill caused asymmetrical splitting (*New York Times, op.cit*).

The latest trend in the generic drug industry is that *brand-name* companies are producing generic versions of their own drugs. Zoloft, for example, which lost patent protection in 2006, is now manufactured as generic sertraline by several companies, including Teva, which is a large pharmaceutical company specializing in generics, and Greenstone, which is a division of Pfizer, the originator of Zoloft.

But wait! Recall that the Hatch-Waxman Act awards the first generic company (in this case, Teva) six months of marketing exclusivity. So why is Pfizer allowed to sell generic sertraline during that period as well? There's no good reason. The original Hatch-Waxman Act didn't foresee that originator companies would ever have any interest in producing generics, and so did not include any language forbidding this practice. This loophole in the law is being exploited by brand name companies who realize how profitable generics can be.

The legality of this trend is being debated in various court rooms. But the implication for clinicians is that the next time a patient calls to complain that his or her subscription was filled as a generic, you can reply that chances are decent that it was produced by the same factory that produced the brand name version he or she used to ingest.

Generic Drugs in Psychiatry:
A Review of the Research

Now that you know more about the generic drug industry, we'll go ahead and review the research on whether certain specific generic psychiatric drugs are as efficacious as their branded cousins.

In general, as you review the research on generics, you'll note that most articles are case reports of patients switched from branded to generic medications. The switch is usually reported as having caused problems, such as new side effects or worsening symptoms (most recently, see Desmarais JE et al, *CNS Neurosci Ther*, 2011;17(6):750–760). If you relied on these studies you'd probably be scared away from ever prescribing a generic again.

Before coming to any rash conclusions, note that case reports are notoriously subject to bias of various kinds. One is recall bias—you are much more likely to remember the few patients who had problems than the majority of patients who did fine. In many cases, you may not even know which of your patients are taking brand vs. generic, since that decision may be made at the pharmacy. Another problem with case reports is a tendency to attribute complications to a generic switch rather than to other factors, such as psychosocial issues, or to a negative placebo effect in which a patient expects to do more poorly if he or she knows a generic switch has been made. Finally, there is sometimes bias caused by financial relationships with pharmaceutical companies that stand to profit from research damning generics.

In order to truly test generics, you should randomly assign patients to continuing on the brand vs. switching, and you should make sure both the doctors and the patients are unaware of which patients are getting which treatment (the so-called randomized double-blind study). To give you an illustration of the progression from inadequate studies to well-designed trials, I'll describe the most well-studied generic in psychiatry—clozapine (brand name, Clozaril).

Soon after generic clozapine came to market in 1999, several case reports appeared describing reemergence of psychotic symptoms after switching from Clozaril to clozapine. Soon, both Novartis (the manufacturer of Clozaril) and generic manufacturers commissioned large studies that compared Clozaril with generic clozapine. The results of these studies depended on the source of funding. There was a neat split between the studies funded by Novartis, which reported that patients switched to generic clozapine did poorly (Kluznik JC et al, *J Clin Psychiatry* 2001;62[suppl 5]:14–17; Mofsen R & Balter J, *Clin Ther* 2001;23(10):1720–1731), and the studies funded by generic companies, which reported that the generic was well-tolerated (Makela EH et al, *Ann Pharmacother* 2003;37(3):350–353; Stoner SC et al, *Pharmacotherapy* 2003;23(6):806–810). The Novartis-funded studies caused a significant ruckus, and the FDA responded by requesting the generic makers to repeat their bioequivalence research, which they did, apparently to the FDA's satisfaction.

More recently, two larger studies have been published without any industry funding—brand company or generic. Both appear to exonerate generic clozapine. The larger of the two was a retrospective study of 337 patients who were switched from Clozaril to generic clozapine. When assessed three months after switching, the majority of patients either had improved clinically (as measured by the Clinical Global Impression) or showed no change (Paton C, *Br J Psychiatry* 2006;189(2):184–185). The other study, also retrospective, followed 58 patients after the Clozaril-to-clozapine switch. At six-month follow-up, the study found no clinical worsening either in terms of psychotic symptoms or in terms of white blood cell counts (Alessi-Severini S et al, *J Clin Psychiatry* 2006;67(7):1047–1054).

Thus, large-scale studies conducted by investigators without commercial conflicts of interest indicate that generic clozapine is as safe and effective as brand name Clozaril.

What about antidepressants? A number of review articles cite a study of six patients who were switched from Prozac to generic fluoxetine; all of these patients experienced adverse events or psychiatric worsening (Yu BP et al, *J Affect Disord* 2004;81(2):185–186). However, this was an uncontrolled case series of a small number of patients, and so may not be representative of the general patient population. In addition, the senior author of this report is a speaker for Eli Lilly, the manufacturer of Prozac, bringing up the possibility that commercial bias may have affected the selection of patients and the rating of adverse events.

Another frequently-cited article is a double-blind crossover study in which patients were assigned to Prozac vs. generic fluoxetine. The authors reported that the generic caused more diarrhea and that Prozac improved depression more robustly (Bakish D et al. A double-blind, crossover study comparing generic and brand fluoxetine in the treatment of major depressive disorder. Poster presented at 40th Annual Meeting of NIMH, New Clinical Drug Evaluation Unit NCDEU; 2000; Boca Raton, FL). But again, there are significant problems in interpreting this report: 1) the lead author is an Eli Lilly speaker, 2) the report has never been published in a peer-reviewed journal, and 3) the generic formulation of fluoxetine used in this study is one that has never been approved for use in the United States.

The only generic antidepressant that has been clearly shown to be inferior to brand was Teva's 300 mg version of GlaxoSmithKline's Wellbutrin XL. In 2007, the FDA received reports of about 78 patients who were switched from Wellbutrin XL 300 mg to Teva Pharmaceutical's generic Budeprion XL 300 mg. The complaints ranged from lack of efficacy to new onset side effects. A private lab called Consumer Lab (http://bit.ly/1zDhHpx) ran its own tests of the generic and found that 34% of the bupropion contained in the pill had been released after two hours, as opposed to only 8% of the bupropion in Wellbutrin XL. The FDA eventually conducted its own bioequivalence study, and found that, indeed, the generic Budeprion XL was not bioequivalent to the brand version, with its Cmax reaching only 75% of the value for Wellbutrin XL. Therefore, the FDA asked Teva to withdraw the 300 mg capsule from the market, which it did. However, Teva's Budeprion XL 150 mg is still available, and there are four other generic versions of Wellbutrin XL (from different companies) that are on the market and for which there are no concerns about bioequivalence. (For a very detailed account of this story see the interesting Q&A on the FDA's website at http://1.usa.gov/14M42To.) The bottom line is that extended-release formulations may be harder for generic companies to accurately copy—though this has been shown to affect only one dose strength of one product.

In terms of research on generic benzodiazepines, there is a published report relevant to the anecdotal impression that generic clonazepam is less effective than branded Klonopin. This report is contained in a letter from a psychiatrist concerning two of his private-practice patients. In both patients, the generic version actually was *more* anxiolytic and sedating than the brand name version, exactly opposite to common opinion (Rapaport MH, *J Clin Psychopharm* 1997;17(5):424).

As opposed to antidepressants and anxiolytics, there is a fair amount of literature on brand vs. generic *anticonvulsants,* but this is limited to its uses for seizure disorder. A meta-analysis of such studies published in 2010 found no differences in clinical outcomes between the two formulations (Kesselheim AS et al, *Drugs* 2010;70(5):605–621). As is often the case in this literature, case reports find that switching to generics leads to problems, but subsequent larger studies report equivalence. For example, some case reports had indicated complications or breakthrough seizures after patients are switched from Tegretol to generic carbamazepine, but two rigorous double-blind comparisons showed no differences in bioavailability or clinical efficacy (Oles KS et al, *Neurology* 1992;42(6):1147–1153; Silpakit O et al, *Ann Pharmacother* 1997;31(5):548–552).

In sum, the published literature on generic psychiatric medications is not robust enough to draw any definitive conclusions. Each reader has likely developed his or her own clinical feeling for which generics are more or less likely to result in patient phone calls, and this may be the best "information" we have at this point.

The Patent-Extension Shuffle: The Case of BuSpar

Whether generics are truly bioequivalent or not, their use has skyrocketed, and income from brand name drugs has dropped precipitously. For that reason, drug companies have gone to great lengths to prevent generic drugs from being approved and have taken advantage of whatever loopholes they can find in order to accomplish this end.

An example of this is BuSpar. BuSpar was initially created by Bristol-Myers Squibb (BMS) in 1980, and therefore it was due for patent expiration in 2000. The generic company Mylan Laboratories had been waiting in the wings for the opportunity to be the first company to produce generic buspirone. BuSpar's patent was set to expire on November 22, 2000, and Mylan's trucks were loading up with crates of generic buspirone the day before.

The trucks never made it to the pharmacies, however, because on November 21, BMS was awarded a *new* patent—for a metabolite of BuSpar, 6-hydroxy-buspirone, which is apparently the active anti-anxiety ingredient of BuSpar. Because of this new patent, Mylan was obliged to challenge its legitimacy in court before it could ship out any generic buspirone. Over the next few months, Mylan's attorneys argued what appears to be an obvious point— namely that the actual medication that patients swallow is buspirone and not the newly discovered metabolite. Mylan was not attempting to market a generic version of the metabolite, but only a generic version of the parent compound, whose patent had clearly expired.

BMS's counter argument was that once any patient swallowed a Mylan generic buspirone, his or her body would create the newly patented metabolite 6-hydroxy-buspirone. At the moment that a patient's liver synthesized that compound, Mylan would be guilty of patent infringement.

Eventually the judge ruled in favor of Mylan, saying that BMS had gone to ridiculous lengths to maintain its BuSpar monopoly and that the drug's patent protection was officially over. Thus, a full six months after generic buspirone should have become available, it was finally shipped. That six months was extremely lucrative for

BMS—worth at least $300 million (an assumption based on reports that it made $700 million on BuSpar in 2000). It's safe to say that BMS recouped its legal fees and then some. (Documentation for the fascinating BuSpar saga can be found in the report "A Primer: Generic Drugs, Patents and the Pharmaceutical Marketplace," by the *National Institute for Health Care Management*, http://www.nihcm.org.)

Patent Extenders: A Growth Industry

Because the pipeline for novel psychotropic medications has been relatively dry, many drug companies resort to "evergreening" their medications—reformulating them in various ways in order to create products that can be patented.

Typical products introduced as a result of evergreening techniques include:

1. Extended-release medication (see Chapter 4 for numerous examples);

2. Purified stereoisomer of a racemic medication (eg, Lexapro is the S-isomer of Celexa);

3. Active metabolites of a medications (eg, Pristiq is the active metabolite of Effexor);

4. New indications for old medications (eg, Silenor is the antidepressant doxepin approved for insomnia); and

5. Combinations of two older medications to create one "new" medication (eg., Symbyax, a combination of olanzapine and fluoxetine).

These tweaked formulations and new indications don't receive a full 20 years of patent protection, by the way—they may get only three to five years, depending on the technique used. But these extra few years can mean a lot money if a company plays its cards right. In conjunction with creating a patent extender, there are certain marketing techniques commonly used by companies to "migrate" prescriptions from the old version of a drug to the new version:

1. The drug company introduces the new formulation at least one year *before* the old formulation goes generic, and it uses this time to accomplish the migration to brand name. Releasing the new version well before the old version goes generic is crucial, because once physicians become comfortable prescribing the generic, they are less likely to be convinced the tweaked version is worth the extra cost.

2. Drug reps stop sampling the old version before it becomes generic, in order to discourage its use.

3. All promotions of the old version cease, and ads and industry-funded continuing medical education programs focus entirely on the advantages of the "novel" formulation. Sometimes the company will go so far as to actually discontinue all production of the older version which forces reliance on the new one (eg, once Namenda XR was released the company discontinued regular Namenda).

4. The drug company often increases the price of the soon-to-go generic version in order to make the higher price of the new version less of a shock to insurance companies.

Some physicians are surprised that these strategies exist, but they shouldn't be. The pharmaceutical industry is arguably the most profitable endeavor in all of business, and companies have perfected the science of turning a profit. Let's hope they spend as much energy on the science of creating novel medications!

Should you prescribe newly approved versions of older medications? There's no one answer to this question, of course. On the next page I've created a table listing recent patent extenders, explaining the nature of the "tweak," and explaining the putative clinical advantages of the new agent. Sometimes the improvements are genuine, if incremental. In other cases, the improvements are so tiny that prescriptions do little more than increase healthcare costs for everybody. Companies rarely fund research comparing their new formulation with the old one, so there is very little solid data to decide which extenders are worth extending to your patients.

Recent Patent-Extenders in Psychiatry

Original drug	New drug	Mechanism of "Tweak"	Putative advantages
Effexor (venlafaxine)	Pristiq (desvenlafaxine)	Active metabolite of Effexor	Easier to dose, fewer drug-drug interactions
Trazodone	Oleptro (trazodone ER)	Extended release	Less sedation
Dextroamphetamine	Vyvanse (lisdexamfetamine)	Metabolic precursor of dextroamphetamine, attached to lysine	Lower risk of abuse
Risperidone	Invega (paliperidone)	Active metabolite of risperidone, and extended release	Fewer drug-drug interactions
Seroquel (quetiapine)	Seroquel XR (quetiapine XR)	Extended release	Once daily dosing, less sedation
Namenda (memantine)	Namenda XR (memantine XR)	Extended release	Once daily dosing
Lamictal (lamotrigine)	Lamictal XR (lamotrigine XR)	Extended release	Once daily dosing

Chapter 10

The Kidney and Psychiatric Medications

Reviewing the kidney is a good exercise for psychiatrists, because the more we understand about its function, the more adept we become at choosing the right medications for each patient. Here are just three examples—you can probably come up with many others:

1. We prescribe lithium, and we have to know something about the kidney to understand why lithium levels are sometimes too high or too low.

2. We treat older folks and other people with reduced kidney function, and we have to know how to understand measures of kidney function and how this relates to any alterations in dosages of medications.

3. Patients often complain of urination problems and wonder if we are causing these problems because of our medication. Knowing something about the kidney helps us to more legitimately explain what's going on in these cases.

A Brief Lesson on the Kidney

The kidney is the body's great alchemist, turning blood into urine. It's composed of about one million nephrons, which are the working units of the organ. The nephron is the place where blood gets transformed into urine.

In each nephron, the real action occurs in a special tuft of capillaries, which is called the "glomerulus." Think of it as a ball of string, in which the string is a long, twisted capillary. This ball sits inside a roundish cup called a Bowman's capsule, and as the heart pumps blood into the glomerulus, a filtrate is forced out of the capillaries and into the capsule. The pores in these capillaries are huge, so that basically everything filters out, including glucose, plasma, and most drugs that we ingest. What stays behind? Blood cells, big proteins, and any drugs that are bound to proteins.

Now, Bowman's capsule is like the basin of a water fountain with a pipe leading out of it. In the kidney, of course, the pipe is not straight but is winding and quite convoluted, leading to some of the more traumatic memories of Physiology 101, in which we were subjected to terms such as "proximal convoluted tubule," "distal convoluted tubule," "collecting ducts," and—horror of horrors—the "loop of Henle." Basically, they are all terms for different sections of one long twisty pipe carrying the filtrate from Bowman's capsule to the ureters, then to the bladder, and finally to the city plumbing.

Altogether, the blood stream causes 180 liters of fluid per day to be filtered into Bowman's capsule and then into the tubules and ducts of the nephrons. That's more than 20 times the volume of blood. Luckily, the kidney has developed a fiendishly clever mechanism for reabsorbing 99% of the fluid, as well as glucose, vitamins, minerals, amino acids, and lots of ions, such as sodium (Na+) and potassium.

How do we reabsorb all this stuff? Mostly, we do it by forcing Na+ ions out of the tubules and back into the blood stream. Water and lots of other solutes passively follow, and, presto, we've gotten most of our blood back. So why have a kidney at all? What's the purpose of this elaborate process of filtering stuff out and then snatching most of it back in? To get rid of normal metabolic waste products, such as urea, but also to get rid of foreign products that we put into our system, such as medications. But how does the kidney prevent medications from getting reabsorbed along with everything else? Mostly by setting up the tubules in such a way that ionic compounds normally cannot pass through the tubule membranes.

The Kidney

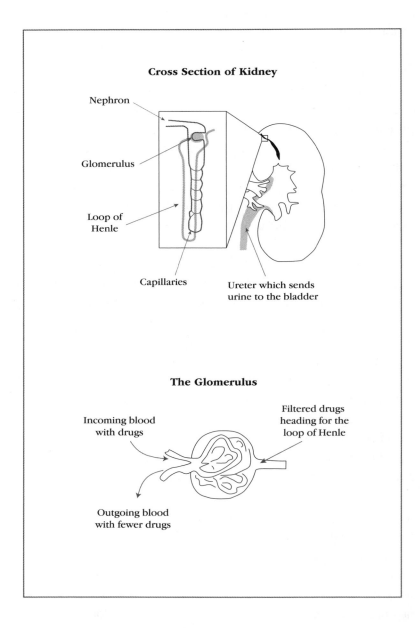

Cross Section of Kidney

Nephron

Glomerulus

Loop of Henle

Capillaries

Ureter which sends urine to the bladder

The Glomerulus

Incoming blood with drugs

Filtered drugs heading for the loop of Henle

Outgoing blood with fewer drugs

Remember in Chapter 5 when we talked about biotransformation? The purpose of that, as you'll recall, was to turn lipophilic drugs into ionic versions of themselves. The ultimate plan was to have these ionic compounds get secreted into the kidney's tubules, and to get trapped there, so that they would exit with the urine.

Lithium and the Kidney

Lithium in the bloodstream travels in its ionic form, Li+, a small molecule similar to Na+. When it reaches the kidney, it gets filtered into Bowman's capsule, and then into the nephron's system of tubules. Ordinarily the Li+ would stay in the tubules and eventually end up in the urine. But if Na+ transporters cannot find enough sodium to reabsorb, they'll sometimes settle for lithium. These are the conditions that lead to toxicity. Here are some of the more common situations:

Dehydration. We're supposed to tell our patients on lithium to guard against dehydration. Why? Because when the kidney senses dehydration, it does what it can to reabsorb water. To accomplish this, it actively reabsorbs lots of Na+, and since Li+ and Na+ look similar to the kidney, it ends up sucking a lot of lithium back into the bloodstream, increasing lithium levels.

Hydrochlorothiazide diuretics. This common diuretic used to treat hypertension acts by increasing sodium excretion in the kidney tubules, leading to increased urination, decreased total body water, and therefore decreased blood pressure. The kidney doesn't particularly like to see such havoc being played with its fine-tuned homeostatic mechanism, and actively tries to compensate for the loss of sodium by retaining it elsewhere in the tubule system. But in snatching back up as much sodium as it can, the kidney indiscriminately snatches up a lot of lithium, causing an increase of up to 40% in lithium levels.

ACE inhibitors. ACE inhibitors (angiotensin-converting-enzyme inhibitors) are also medications used to treat hypertension. They work by inhibiting the formation of angiotensin II, which is normally a vasoconstrictor. If there is less AG-II around, arteries do not constrict as much, and blood pressure is reduced. And how is this related to lithium? AG-II also promotes the release of a hormone called aldosterone, whose function is to cause the kidney to retain sodium. Since ACE inhibitors lower AG-II, they indirectly lower aldosterone, which in turn decreases the kidney's ability to retain sodium. The kidney compensates for this by trying to reabsorb sodium in other parts of the nephron, but it confuses lithium for sodium, causing higher levels of lithium—elevations in the range of 200% to 300%.

NSAIDs. NSAIDs can cause 30% to 60% increases in lithium levels via unclear mechanisms, possibly due to the inhibition of prostaglandins leading to interference with lithium excretion. This includes ibuprofen, Indocin (indomethacin), naproxen, the Cox-2 inhibitor Celebrex (celecoxib), but does not include aspirin and Clinoril (sulindac). In general, for patients vulnerable to this effect, you can expect lithium levels to increase over five to 10 days after adding an NSAID, with levels returning back to baseline again within about seven days (Demler TL, *US Pharm* 2012;37(11):HS16–HS19).

One common dietary constituent can cause **decreased** lithium level—caffeine. Caffeine increases the glomerular filtration rate, causing us to urinate more, leading to indiscriminate losses of solutes. There are cases of patients becoming manic after increasing caffeine intake, not because of the caffeine itself but because the caffeine significantly decreased their lithium levels. (See two such cases in *Drug-Drug Interaction Primer: A Compendium of Case Vignettes for the Practicing Clinician* by Neil Sandson (Arlington VA: American Psychiatic Publishing; 2007).

Does Lithium Damage the Kidney?

In Chapter 4 we discussed the evidence that once daily dosing of lithium might lead to less polyuria than multiple dosing. Polyuria *per se* is not tantamount to kidney damage, but it is certainly an irritating side effect that our patients would prefer not to have.

In terms of actual kidney damage, it turns out that about 10% to 20% of patients on long-term lithium treatment experience some degree of renal insufficiency, defined by most of the studies that have looked at this as an increase in serum creatinine. The most recent study examined 114 psychiatric outpatients who had been taking lithium continuously for at least four years. Twenty four (21%) of these patients exhibited the "creeping creatinine" phenomenon, with levels gradually reaching the 1.5 level, which is the standard cutoff point for renal impairment. Most of these patients did not show this sign of renal impairment until 10 to 15 years into lithium treatment (Lepkifker E et al, *J Clin Psychiatry* 2004;65(7):850–856).

The positive spin on these findings is that the majority of patients on long-term lithium treatment showed no signs of renal impairment whatsoever. In addition, in half of the patients with renal problems, the creatinine elevations reversed with simple dosage reductions.

The bottom line here is to monitor creatinine levels on a regular basis (twice a year or so) in your lithium patients, and to continue this regular monitoring no matter how long your patient has been on this medication.

Assuming that your patient is experiencing polyuria without increased creatinine, what he is suffering from is termed "lithium-induced diabetes insipidus," a condition in which lithium disrupts the concentrating ability of the collecting tubules. A normal amount of urine per day is about 1.5 liters, and polyuria is defined as more than two to 2.5 liters per day.

Oddly, the way to treat patients who have severe polyuria and who need to remain on lithium is to give them a potassium-sparing diuretic, a medication that is usually used to increase urine production. How does this paradoxical remedy work? Basically, the diuretics start in the usual way, by limiting sodium reabsorption, thereby increasing urine volume. The body then notices that it has less fluid in it, and this reduces the pressure at the glomerulus, causing a lower glomerular filtration rate. The kidney then responds to this by saying "uh oh, we're running low on fluid, we'd better decrease urine output," leading, finally, to the desired outcome of less polyuria. The best diuretic to use is the potassium-sparing diuretic Midamor (amiloride), dosed at 20 mg QD (Battle DC et al, *N Engl J Med* 1985; 312(7):408–414). It works within three weeks, but it can cause an increase in lithium levels, so you should monitor levels more frequently than usual (every two weeks) when starting or increasing amiloride.

Chapter 11

Pharmacogenetic Testing: Is it Useful in Your Practice?

Keeping track of various drug-drug interactions is hard enough. Now, in order to add another layer of complexity to your daily clinical chores, companies are marketing new pharmacogenetic testing products, which theoretically help us improve our prescribing decisions. In this chapter I'll review the concepts driving these tests as well as the research on whether, at the end of the day, they are actually clinically useful. The available tests measure genes responsible for two kinds of drug effects: pharmacodynamic effects and pharmacokinetic effects. I'll focus on pharmacokinetics, since the tests are most established for this area.

What is P450 Polymorphism?

Just to review our molecular biology: Enzymes are proteins, which are made up of amino acids. Amino acids, in turn, are put together according to the sequences of nucleotide base pairs in our DNA. A "gene" refers to a specific sequence of nucleotide base pairs leading to the formation of a specific compound.

Each of the P450 enzymes is built by a particular gene. Individuals vary in their genetic makeup, and this variability doesn't end with obvious characteristics like eye color and height. In fact, there is inter-individual variability, or "polymorphism," in the genes coding for P450 enzymes.

To understand P450 polymorphisms though, you have to recall

that our chromosomes (the carriers of our genes) come in pairs. As an example, the gene coding for the P450 2D6 enzyme is carried on our 22nd chromosome. Most people have two normal copies of the 2D6 gene—one on each of their copies of chromosome 22. This allows each copy to produce the enzyme, ensuring that we have a good supply and are able to biotransform substrates of 2D6 at the expected rate. Confusingly, the accepted jargon refers to these people as **"extensive metabolizers"** rather than "normal metabolizers."

"Intermediate metabolizers" have one copy of the 2D6 gene, causing them to metabolize drugs a little more slowly than normal. However, there is controversy about whether we should really be concerned about this category, which encompasses about 40% of Caucasians and is similar for most other populations. It isn't clear at this point that dosage adjustments are really necessary in intermediate metabolizers.

"Poor metabolizers," on the other hand, do not have the 2D6 gene on either of their two chromosomes. When given a medication dependent on 2D6 for metabolism, they will have many side effects, because of excessive medication blood levels. Eventually, they are able to eliminate the drug via other enzymes, but it takes a long time. These are likely to be those patients whose charts are filled with lists of drugs that they've tried and discontinued. About 7% to 10% of most populations are poor metabolizers, but for Asians the figure is 1%.

On the other side of the spectrum are **"ultrarapid metabolizers,"** people who have extra copies of the 2D6 gene on one or both chromosome. They manufacture much more 2D6 than most people, so that they metabolize 2D6 substrates at a high rate. These patients need higher-than-standard doses of drugs.

Is P450 Polymorphism Really Clinically Significant?

While there's no question that poor metabolizers and ultrarapid metabolizers exist, there are two questions that need to be answered before we can conclude that testing for these genes is worthwhile. First, does metabolizer status actually affect clinical outcome in real world psychiatric settings? And, second, assuming that P450 poly-phormisms are clinically relevant, do the tests currently available actually lead clinicians to make better prescribing decisions that trans-late to better outcomes for patients?

In terms of the basic question about whether metabolizer status can effect response to meds, there is fairly convincing evi-dence that it does. In one study, 100 consecutive inpatients at a psychiatric hospital were given P450 genotype testing. The ultrar-apid metabolizers (UMs) had the fewest side effects, while the poor metabolizers (PMs) had the most side effects (Chou WH et al, *J Clin Psychopharmacol* 2000;20(2):246–251). In this study, patients who were PMs or UMs specifically for drugs metabolized by the 2D6 enzyme tended to stay in the hospital longer and incurred higher costs, presumably due to the fact that more time was required to adjust dosages prior to discharge.

In another study, also of hospitalized patients, those who were PMs for 2D6 were over three times more likely to have required a switch of antidepressants than normal extensive metaboliz-ers (EMs). Evidently, PMs reported more side effects, leading to changes in medications (Mulder H et al, *J Clin Psychopharmacol* 2005;25(2):188–191). A study with a similar design focused on anti-psychotic drugs and found that PMs were more than four times more likely to require antiparkinsonian medication than EMs (Schillevoort I et al, *Pharmacogenetics* 2002;12(3):235–240).

Does Genetic Testing Improve Your Prescribing Decisions?

Retrospective evidence that metabolizer status might affect response to meds is nice, but the key question is whether ordering genetic tests for a patient will affect your prescribing decisions in a positive way. Answering this question requires more complicated and expensive research. You have to randomly assign patients to testing vs. no testing, and then you have to follow them over a sig-nificant period of time to see if testing makes a difference.

The bottom line is that there is not yet convincing evidence that pharmacogenetic testing is valuable. Let's go quickly through the evidence separated out by diagnosis.

Antidepressants and mood stabilizers. In 2007, the federal government funded a comprehensive review of whether genetic testing improves outcomes for patients taking SSRIs for major depression, one of the most common scenarios in psychiatry. The only consistent finding is that in healthy individuals who take a single dose of an SSRI, metabolizer status significantly predicts the blood levels of SSRIs. However, in studies of real patients taking maintenance doses, there is no clear association. Nor is there an association between metabolizer status and clinical response. Finally, no study has been conducted to assess whether genetic testing guides clinicians in making SSRI prescribing decisions that affect subsequent patient outcomes. The lack of evidence led the group to conclude that "there is insufficient evidence on clinical validity and utility to support a recommendation for or against use of CYP450 testing in adults beginning SSRI treatment for nonpsychotic depression" (Evaluation of Genomic Applications in Practice and Prevention (EGAPP) Working Group, *Genet Med* 2007;9(12):819–825). A more recent review in 2013 concluded that no new studies had been published supporting such testing since the 2007 paper was published (Lage G, *CNS Spectrums* 2013;18(5):272–284).

More broadly, it appears that there is no consensus that genetic testing is helpful for the treatment of any mood disorder, including major depression or bipolar disorder, with one exception: Tegretol. Certain patients of Asian ancestry are at high risk of developing Stevens-Johnson syndrome, a dangerous rash in which the skin peels off. In order to determine this risk, the FDA recommends ordering a test for the HLA-B*1502 allele. If patients test positive for this, you should either not use Tegretol, or use it very cautiously.

Antipsychotics. The most recent review of the pharmacogenetics of antipsychotics concluded that there is still no consensus on the utility of genetic testing, with the exception of the first generation antipsychotic Orap (Brandl EJ et al, *Can J Psychiatry* 2014;59(2):76–88). Before prescribing this antipsychotic, you should get CYP2D6 testing. Patients who are poor metabolizers should not take Orap because of the risk of QT prolongation and cardiac arrhythmias.

Bottom Line:
For Whom Should You Order P450 Genotyping?

As reviewed previously, there are really only two clinical situations in psychiatry in which genetic testing is mandatory:

1. Order an HLA-B*1502 test in Asians before prescribing Tegretol.

2. Order a CYP2D6 test in all patients before prescribing Orap.

Beyond these situations, some clinicians may look at the evidence and decide that testing for metabolizer status for various P450 enzymes is potentially helpful. Potential reasons to do this include the following:

1. Patients who are taking multiple medications. For example, if a patient is taking Prozac and Risperdal, there may well be a drug interaction in which Prozac increases Risperdal levels by inhibiting 2D6. This effect might be aggravated further if a patient is a poor metabolizer of 2D6. In such a case, determining metabolizer status might be reasonable, though a more conservative approach would be to simply switch the patient to an alternative antipsychotic that is metabolized differently, such as Geodon.

2. Patients who have a history of intolerable side effects to a variety of medications. If patients are poor metabolizers of drugs processed by particular enzymes, testing may provide some guidance in your future prescribing decisions—though remember that prospective studies have not yet shown that this information ultimately yields better outcomes.

3. Patients who consistently do not respond to robust doses of medications. Poor response may be caused by ultrarapid metabolism, which would prompt you to consider starting such patients at higher doses, titrating to higher than usual doses, or choosing an agent with a different metabolic pathway.

Appendix

Tables and Charts

Half-Lives of Psychiatric Medications

Medication	Half-Life (in hours, except where indicated)	Time to Steady State or Elimination
Anti-Anxiety		
BuSpar	2 hours	10 hours
Ativan, Xanax	10 hours	2 days
Klonopin, Valium	40 hours	8 days
Sleeping Pills		
Sonata	1 hour	5 hours
Ambien	2.5 hours	12 hours
Lunesta	6 hours	30 hours
Restoril, Trazodone	10 hours	2 days
Antidepressants		
Effexor	6 hours	30 hours
Parnate	2.5 hours	12 hours
Cymbalta, Fetzima (levomilnacipran), Nardil, Pristiq	12 hours	3 days
Celexa, Clomipramine, Desipramine, Emsam, Lexapro, Paxil, Remeron, Wellbutrin, Viibryd, Zoloft	24 hours	5 days
Nortriptyline	36 hours	8 days
Vortioxetine (Brintellix)	3 days	15 days
Prozac	10–14 days	50 days
Mood Stabilizers		
Depakote	10 hours	2 days
Tegretol	24 hours initially, then 15 hours after auto-induction	3 days
Lithium, Lamictal	24 hours	5 days

Continued on next page

Half-Lives of Psychiatric Medications
(continued)

Medication	Half-Life (in hours, except where indicated)	Time to Steady State or Elimination
Antipsychotics		
Seroquel, Geodon	6 hours	30 hours
Clozaril, Trilafon	10 hours	2 days
Fanapt, Haldol, Invega, Latuda, Risperdal, Saphris, Zyprexa	24 hours	5 days
Abilify	3 days	15 days
PDE5 Inhibitors		
Levitra, Stendra (avanafil), Viagra	4 hours	1 day
Cialis	18 hours	4 days

Note: Half-life figures derive from a variety of sources, including drug package inserts, textbooks, and online databases. These figures are all *approximate*, and wide variations in half-life estimates are often published, depending on the pharmacokinetic studies referenced.

Psychiatric Drug Interactions by Medication

Medication	Substrate of	Potently Inhibits	Potently Induces	Red Flags*
Antidepressants				
Amitriptyline (Elavil)	2C19, 2D6, 3A4	None	None	Increased by various 2D6 inhibitors
Bupropion (Wellbutrin)	2B6	2D6	None	Increased venlafaxine
Citalopram (Celexa)	2C19, 2D6, 3A4	None	None	No red flags
Clomipramine (Anafranil)	2C19, 2D6	2D6	None	Increased by various 2D6 inhibitors
Desipramine (Norpramin)	2D6	None	None	Increased by various 2D6 inhibitors
Desvenlafaxine (Pristiq)	UGT, 3A4	None	None	No red flags
Duloxetine (Cymbalta)	1A2, 2D6	2D6	None	Increases tricyclics
Escitalopram (Lexapro)	2C19, 2D6, 3A4	None	None	No red flags
Fluoxetine (Prozac)	2D6	2C19, 2D6	None	Increases tricyclics, risperidone
Fluvoxamine (Luvox)	1A2, 2D6	1A2, 2C9, 2C19, 3A4	None	Increases clomipramine, thioridazine, clozapine, olanzapine
Levomilnacipran (Fetzima)	3A4	None	None	No red flags
MAOIs	Not well known	None	None	Dietary; serotonergic; sympathomimetic agents
Mirtazapine (Remeron)	1A2, 2D6, 3A4	None	None	No red flags

*The "red flags" column is reserved for drug combinations that are likely to cause significant and clinically serious drug interactions. It's not comprehensive, and you'll see many less serious potential interactions missing. To find all possible interactions, use software such as Epocrates, or cross-check this table with our table, "Psychiatric Drug Interactions by Enzyme Family."

Continued on next page

Psychiatric Drug Interactions by Medication *(continued)*

Medication	Substrate of	Potently Inhibits	Potently Induces	Red Flags*
Antidepressants *(continued)*				
Nefazodone (Serzone)	3A4	3A4	None	Contraindicated with pimozide
Nortriptyline (Pamelor)	2C19, 3A4	None	None	Increased by various ADs
Paroxetine (Paxil)	2D6	2D6	None	Increases tricyclics, risperidone
Selegiline patch (EMSAM)	2B6	None	None	Usual MAOI cautions
Sertraline (Zoloft)	2C19, 2D6, 3A4	2D6 (≥150mg/d), glucuronidation	None	Increases lamotrigine, tricyclics
St. John's wort	Unclear	None	1A2, 2C9, 3A4, P-glycoprotein	Decreases indinavir, birth control pill
Trazodone (Oleptro)	3A4	None	p-glycoprotein	No red flags
Venlafaxine (Effexor)	2D6, 3A4	None	None	Increased by bupropion
Vilazodone (Viibryd)	3A4	None	None	No red flags
Vortioxetine (Brintellix)	2D6	None	None	No red flags

*The "red flags" column is reserved for drug combinations that are likely to cause significant and clinically serious drug interactions. It's not comprehensive, and you'll see many less serious potential interactions missing. To find all possible interactions, use software such as Epocrates, or cross-check this table with our table, "Psychiatric Drug Interactions by Enzyme Family."

Continued on next page

Psychiatric Drug Interactions by Medication *(continued)*

Medication	Substrate of	Potently Inhibits	Potently Induces	Red Flags*
Antipsychotics				
Aripiprazole (Abilify)	2D6, 3A4	None	None	Increased by various ADs; decreased by carbamazepine (CBZ)
Asenapine (Saphris)	1A2, glucuronidation	2D6	None	Avoid food or drink for 10 minutes after taking
Clozapine (Clozaril)	1A2, 2D6, 3A4	None	None	Decreased by smoking
Haloperidol (Haldol)	2D6	2D6	None	Increased by various ADs
Iloperidone (Fanapt)	2D6, 3A4	None	None	Increased by 2D6, 3A4 inhibitors
Lurasidone (Latuda)	3A4	None	None	No red flags
Olanzapine (Zyprexa)	1A2, glucuronidation	None	None	Increased by fluvoxamine; decreased by smoking, CBZ
Paliperidone (Invega)	misc. non-P450	None	None	No red flags
Perphenazine (Trilafon)	2D6	2D6	None	No red flags
Quetiapine (Seroquel)	3A4	None	None	No red flags
Risperidone (Risperdal)	2D6, 3A4	None	None	Increased by various ADs; decreased by CBZ
Ziprasidone (Geodon)	3A4, misc. non-P450	None	None	Contraindicated with various drugs that cause QT widening

Continued on next page

*The "red flags" column is reserved for drug combinations that are likely to cause significant and clinically serious drug interactions. It's not comprehensive, and you'll see many less serious potential interactions missing. To find all possible interactions, use software such as Epocrates, or cross-check this table with our table, "Psychiatric Drug Interactions by Enzyme Family."

Psychiatric Drug Interactions by Medication (continued)

Medication	Substrate of	Potently Inhibit	Potently Induces	Red Flags*
Anxiolytics/Hypnotics				
Alprazolam (Xanax)	3A4	None	None	No red flags
Buspirone (BuSpar)	3A4	None	None	No red flags
Clonazepam (Klonopin)	3A4	None	None	No red flags
Diazepam (Valium)	2C19, 3A4	None	None	No red flags
Doxepin (Silenor)	2D6	None	None	Increased by 2D6 inhibitors
Eszopiclone (Lunesta)	3A4	None	None	No red flags
Lorazepam (Ativan)	Glucuronidation	None	None	No red flags
Melatonin	1A2	1A2 possibly	None	No red flags
Oxazepam (Serax)	Glucuronidation	None	None	No red flags
Pregabalin (Lyrica)	None	None	None	No red flags
Ramelteon (Rozerem)	1A2	None	None	No red flags
Temazepam (Restoril)	Glucuronidation	None	None	No red flags
Triazolam (Halcion)	3A4	None	None	No red flags
Zaleplon (Sonata)	3A4	None	None	No red flags
Zolpidem (Ambien)	3A4	None	None	No red flags

*The "red flags" column is reserved for drug combinations that are likely to cause significant and clinically serious drug interactions. It's not comprehensive, and you'll see many less serious potential interactions missing. To find all possible interactions, use software such as Epocrates, or cross-check this table with our table, "Psychiatric Drug Interactions by Enzyme Family."

Continued on next page

Psychiatric Drug Interactions by Medication *(continued)*

Medication	Substrate of	Potently Inhibits	Potently Induces	Red Flags*
Dementia Medications				
Donepezil (Aricept)	2D6, 3A4	None	None	Caution with anticholinergics, beta blockers
Galantamine (Razadyne)	2D6, 3A4	None	None	Caution with anticholinergics, beta blockers
Memantine (Namenda)	non-P450	None	None	No red flags
Rivastigmine (Exelon)	non-P450	None	None	Caution with anticholinergics, beta blockers
Mood Stabilizers				
Carbamazepine (Tegretol, Equetro)	3A4	None	1A2, 3A4, glucuronidation	No red flags
Divalproex (Depakote)	Glucuronidation	Glucuronidation	None	Increases lamotrigine
Gabapentin (Neurontin)	Excreted unchanged	None	None	No red flags
Lamotrigine (Lamictal)	Glucuronidation	None	None	Increased by divalproex; decreased by estrogen
Lithium (Lithobid, Eskalith)	Renal elimination	None	None	Increased by NSAIDs, ACE inhibitors, diuretics (see Chapter 10)
Oxcarbazepine (Trileptal)	Phase II	2C19	3A4 (milder than CBZ), glucuronidation	Decreases birth control pills
Topiramate (Topamax)	Mostly unchanged	None	Unclear	Decreases birth control pills

*The "red flags" column is reserved for drug combinations that are likely to cause significant and clinically serious drug interactions. It's not comprehensive, and you'll see many less serious potential interactions missing. To find all possible interactions, use software such as Epocrates, or cross-check this table with our table, "Psychiatric Drug Interactions by Enzyme Family."

Continued on next page

Psychiatric Drug Interactions by Medication *(continued)*

Medication	Substrate of	Potently Inhibits	Potently Induces	Red Flags*
Others				
Atomoxetine (Strattera)	2D6, 2C19	None	None	No red flags
Caffeine	1A2	None	None	Decreases Lithium (by diuresis)
Grapefruit Juice	NA	3A4	None	Increases multiple medications
Guanfacine	3A4	None	None	No red flags
Modafinil (Provigil)	3A4	None	3A4 (milder than CBZ)	Decreases birth control pills
PDE5 Inhibitors Avanafil (Stendra) Sildenafil (Viagra) Tadalafil (Cialis) Vardenafil (Levitra)	3A4	None	None	Contraindicated with. nitrates;caution with alpha blockers
Psychostimulants	Complex metabolism	None	None	No red flags
Smoking	NA	None	1A2	Decreases clozapine and olanzapine

*The "red flags" column is reserved for drug combinations that are likely to cause significant and clinically serious drug interactions. It's not comprehensive, and you'll see many less serious potential interactions missing. To find all possible interactions, use software such as Epocrates, or cross-check this table with our table, "Psychiatric Drug Interactions by Enzyme Family."

Psychiatric Drug Interactions by Enzyme Family

P450 Family	Inhibitors	Inducers	Substrates	
			Psychiatric	*Non-Psychiatric*
3A4	**Grapefruit juice** **Fluoxetine** **Fluvoxamine** **Nefazodone**	**Modafinil** **Tegretol** *Next 3 less significant:* **St. John's wort** **Oxcarbazepine** **Topiramate**	**Eszopiclone, Zolpidem, Ramelteon, Zaleplon** (Ind: lack of hypnotic efficacy) **Buspirone** (Inh: N/V, dizziness, sedation) **Methadone** (Inh: sedation, miosis; Ind: opioid withdrawal) **Carbamazepine** (Inh: fatigue, confusion; Ind: breakthrough seizures) **Tricyclics** (Inh: sedation, arrhythmias) **Alprazolam** (Inh: sedation)	**Birth control pills** (Ind: pregnancy) **Calcium channel blockers** (Inh: hypotension) **Cyclosporine** (Ind: transplant rejection) **Statins** (Inh: ↑ LFTs, rhabdomyolysis)
2D6	**Asenapine** **Duloxetine** **Haloperidol** **Fluoxetine** **Paroxetine** **Perphenazine** **Sertraline (≥150mg/day)** *Next 2 less significant:* **Bupropion** **Tricyclics**	No Inducers!	**Duloxetine** **Tricyclics** **Venlafaxine**	**Beta blockers** (Inh: hypotension) **Hydrocodone** (Inh: pro-drug—less analgesia) **Tramadol** (Inh: pro-drug—less analgesia)

Continued on next page

Key: "Inh" = inhibition; "Ind" = induction; "N/V" = nausea/vomiting; "pro-drug" means that parent compound is metabolized into the active agent; in these cases, inhibition leads to less drug activity.

Psychiatric Drug Interactions by Enzyme Family *(continued)*

P450 Family	Inhibitors	Inducers	Substrates	
			Psychiatric	**Non-Psychiatric**
1A2	Fluvoxamine	Carbamazepine (mild) Smoking St. John's wort	**Asenapine** **Caffeine** (Inh: jittery) **Clozapine** (Inh: orthostasis, sedation) **Duloxetine** **Fluvoxamine** **Melatonin** **Mirtazapine** **Olanzapine** (Inh: sedation, constipation; Ind: decompensation) **Ramelteon**	None of great significance
2C9	Fluvoxamine St. John's wort	No significant inducers	None of great significance	**Oral Hypoglycemics** (Inh: low blood sugar) Warfarin
2B6	None	No significant inducers	Bupropion Selegiline	None of great significance
2C19	Fluoxetine Fluvoxamine Oxcarbazetine	St. John's wort	Citalopram Escitalopram Sertraline Tricyclics	None of great significance
Protein Binding	Fluoxetine Paroxetine Prozac Sertraline Valproic acid	No significant inducers	None of great significance	**Digoxin** (Inh: arrhythmia, N/V, confusion) **Phenytoin** (Inh: confusion, ataxia) **Warfarin** (Inh: ↑ PT, bruising, bleeding)
Miscellaneous	**Valproic acid** increases levels of Lamictal **Thioridazine** is contraindicated with Luvox, Paxil, and Prozac **Fluvoxamine** increases levels of Haldol			

Key: "Inh" = inhibition; "Ind" = induction; "N/V" = nausea/vomiting; "pro-drug" means that parent compound is metabolized into the active agent; in these cases, inhibition leads to less drug activity.

Common Non-Psychiatric Meds and Their Interactions

Medication	Significant Interactions with Psychiatric Drugs
Anti-Infectives	
Amoxicillin	None
Azithromycin (Zithromax)	Contraindicated with pimozide; caution with ziprasidone
Cephalosporins (eg, Keflex)	None
Ciprofloxacin clarithromycin erythromycin ketoconazole	Increases zolpidem, buspirone, clozapine, methadone, carbamazepine, diazepam, alprazolam; contraindicated with pimozide
Levofloxacin (Levaquin)	Contraindicated with pimozide
Asthma	
Albuterol (Ventolin HFA)	MAOIs and tricylics use with caution
Fluticasone propionate and salmeterol (Advair Diskus)	MAOIs and tricylics use with caution: level increases with fluvoxamine
Tiotropium bromide (Spiriva Handihaler)	Caution with anticholingerics
Cardiac Meds	
Amlodipine (Norvasc)	None
Atorvastatin (Lipitor)	Level increased by fluoxetine
Clopidogrel (Plavix)	None
Digox (Lanoxin)	Level decreased by St. John's wort
Diltiazem (Cardizem)	Increases buspirone, carbamazepine, triazolam, midazolam
Enalapril (Vasotec)	None
Ezetimibe (Zetia)	None
Furosemide (Lasix)	None
Hydrochlorothiazide	Increases lithium
Lisinopril (Zestril)	Increases lithium
Nifedipine (Procardia)	None

Continued on next page

Common Non-Psychiatric Meds and
Their Interactions *(continued)*

Medication	Significant Interactions with Psychiatric Drugs
Cardiac Meds (continued)	
Pravastatin (Pravachol)	None
Quinidine (Quinidex)	Level increased by fluvoxamine, nefazodone
Rosuvastatin calcium (Crestor)	None
Simvastatin (Zocor)	Level increased by fluoxetine
Valsartan (Diovan)	Increases lithium
Verapamil (Calan)	Increases buspirone, carbamazepine, triazolam, midazolam
Warfarin (Coumadin)	Level increased by fluvoxamine, fluoxetine
Diabetes Meds	
Glipizide (Glucotrol)	Level increased by divalproex
Glyburide	None
Insulin	None
Insulin (Lantus Solostar)	MAOIs may increase insulin
Metformin	None
Pioglitazone (Actos)	None
Rosiglitazone (Avandia)	None
Sitagliptin (Januvia)	None
GI Meds	
Antacids (OTC)	None
Cimetidine (Tagamet)	Increases alprazolam, clozapine, paroxetine, fluoxetine, olanzapine, and others
Esomeprazole (Nexium)	None
Lansoprazole (Prevacid)	None
Omeprazole (Prilosec)	Increases diazepam, carbamazepine
Pantoprazole (Protonix)	None
Ranitidine (Zantac)	None

Continued on next page

Common Non-Psychiatric Meds and
Their Interactions (continued)

Medication	Significant Interactions with Psychiatric Drugs
Pain Meds	
Aspirin (Bayer)	Increases divalproex
Acetaminophen (Tylenol)	None
Celecoxib (Celebrex)	Increased by paroxetine, fluoxetine
Codeine	None
Hydrocodone (Vicodin)	Paroxetine, fluoxetine decrease efficacy
Ibuprofen (Advil)	None
Methadone	Level decreased by carbamazepine; level increased by fluvoxamine; increases desipramine
Oxycodone (OxyContin)	None
Oxycodone (Percocet)	None
Sumatriptan (Imitrex)	Possible serotonin syndrome
Tramadol (Ultram)	Paroxetine, fluoxetine decrease efficacy
Others	
Adalimumab (Humira)	None
Cyclobenzaprine (Flexeril)	Contraindicated with MAOIs
Etanercept (Enbrel)	None
Infliximab (Remicade)	None
Levothyroxine	None
Oral Contraceptives	Level decreased by carbamazepine, St. John's wort, modafinil, oxcarbazepine, topiramate; decreases lamotrigine
Tamsulosin (Flomax)	Increased by nefazodone
Tolterodine (Detrol)	None

Annotated
(and Opinionated)
Bibliography

There are some fantastic books out there, and here is a list of my favorites, all of which I relied upon heavily in researching and writing this book.

Wynn GH, Oesterheld JR, Cozza KL, Armstrong SC. *Clinical Manual of Drug Interaction Principles for Medical Practice.* Arlington, VA: American Psychiatric Publishing; 2008.
Part of the "Clinical Manual" series, this book serves as an adequate reference book for almost all your drug interaction information needs.

Katzung B, Trevor A. *Basic and Clinical Pharmacology, 13th ed.* New York: McGraw-Hill Education; 2015.
More manageable and to-the-point than that old standard, Goodman and Gilman.

Puzantian T, Balt S. *Medication Fact Book for Psychiatric Practice, 2nd edition.* Newburyport, MA: Carlat Publishing; 2014.
This spiral-bound book includes medication fact sheets that provide in-depth prescribing information for select psychiatric medications, as well as quick-scan medication tables.

2015 Physician's Desk Reference, 69th ed. Montvale, NJ: PDR Network; 2015.
This huge tome still covers the landscape of drug pharmacoki- netics better than anything else out there. Not suitable for beach reading.

Pronsky ZM, Crowe J. *Food-Medication Interactions, 17th ed.* Birchrunville, PA: Food Medication Interactions; 2012.

Talk about a diamond in the rough! This little spiral-bound book, now in its 17th edition, provides an alphabetical list of every medication out there, and tells you how food affects it, how the drug affects the GI system, and many more useful tidbits.

Sandson NB. *Drug-Drug Interaction Primer: A Compendium of Case Vignettes for the Practicing Clinician.* Arlington, VA: American Psychiatric Publishing; 2007.

Okay, I'll admit to being a Neil Sandson groupie. You'll join the club, too, after reading this book. Sandson builds on an earlier work, and includes over 170 case vignettes illustrating important drug interactions, indexed in multiple clever ways, and written extremely well.

The Carlat Psychiatry Report (monthly newsletter). Newburyport, MA: Carlat Publishing.

Shameless self promotion? I plead guilty.

Walsh CT, Schwartz-Bloom RD. *Levine's Pharmacology: Drug Actions and Reactions, 7th ed.* Boca Raton, FL: CRC Press; 2004.

A wonderfully written, though very detailed, textbook that actually explains all the intricacies of pharmacokinetics and pharmacodynamics in such a way that you will understand them in your bones.

Index

Notes:

1. While almost all current psychiatric medications are mentioned in the text, only those that are discussed at some length are listed in the index. If a medication of interest is not in the index, chances are that you will find it in one of the charts in the Appendix which begins on page 119.

2. Medications are listed in the index under their *trade* names rather than their generic names, in order to make it easier to find relevant information more quickly.

Xanax, 23, 28, 31, 35, 54, 56, 120, 125
Xanax XR, 28, 35
Ziprasidone. *See Geodon*

Notes

Notes

Notes

Notes

Notes

Notes